Pain Management – Research and Technology

NECK PAIN

CAUSES, DIAGNOSIS AND MANAGEMENT

Pain Management - Research and Technology

Additional books in this series can be found on Nova's website under the Series tab.

Additional E-books in this series can be found on Nova's website under the E-book tab.

Pain Management -- Research and Technology

NECK PAIN

CAUSES, DIAGNOSIS AND MANAGEMENT

GREGORIO LOMBARDI
EDITOR

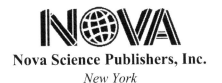

Nova Science Publishers, Inc.
New York

Copyright © 2012 by Nova Science Publishers, Inc.

All rights reserved. No part of this book may be reproduced, stored in a retrieval system or transmitted in any form or by any means: electronic, electrostatic, magnetic, tape, mechanical photocopying, recording or otherwise without the written permission of the Publisher.

For permission to use material from this book please contact us:
Telephone 631-231-7269; Fax 631-231-8175
Web Site: http://www.novapublishers.com

NOTICE TO THE READER

The Publisher has taken reasonable care in the preparation of this book, but makes no expressed or implied warranty of any kind and assumes no responsibility for any errors or omissions. No liability is assumed for incidental or consequential damages in connection with or arising out of information contained in this book. The Publisher shall not be liable for any special, consequential, or exemplary damages resulting, in whole or in part, from the readers' use of, or reliance upon, this material. Any parts of this book based on government reports are so indicated and copyright is claimed for those parts to the extent applicable to compilations of such works.

Independent verification should be sought for any data, advice or recommendations contained in this book. In addition, no responsibility is assumed by the publisher for any injury and/or damage to persons or property arising from any methods, products, instructions, ideas or otherwise contained in this publication.

This publication is designed to provide accurate and authoritative information with regard to the subject matter covered herein. It is sold with the clear understanding that the Publisher is not engaged in rendering legal or any other professional services. If legal or any other expert assistance is required, the services of a competent person should be sought. FROM A DECLARATION OF PARTICIPANTS JOINTLY ADOPTED BY A COMMITTEE OF THE AMERICAN BAR ASSOCIATION AND A COMMITTEE OF PUBLISHERS.

Additional color graphics may be available in the e-book version of this book.

Library of Congress Cataloging-in-Publication Data

Neck pain : causes, diagnosis, and management / editor, Gregorio Lombardi.
   p. ; cm.
 Includes bibliographical references and index.
 ISBN 978-1-61470-363-1 (hardcover)
 1. Neck pain--Etiology. 2. Neck pain--Treatment. 3. Neck pain--Diagnosis. I. Lombardi, Gregorio.
 [DNLM: 1. Neck Pain--etiology. 2. Neck--physiology. 3. Neck Pain--diagnosis. 4. Neck Pain--therapy. WE 708]
 RC936.N44 2011
 612.7'6--dc23
                   2011022208

Published by Nova Science Publishers, Inc. † New York

CONTENTS

Preface		vii
Chapter 1	Cervical Facet Joint Pain: Biomechanics, Neuroanatomy and Neurophysiology *Haibin Chen, Liying Zhang, Zhengguo Wang, John Michael Cavanaugh and King H. Yang*	1
Chapter 2	Work-Related Musculoskeletal Discomfort in the Neck Due to Computer Use *Orhan Korhan*	17
Chapter 3	Support of RSI: Rolfing Structural Integration for Reducing Pain and Limitations of Motion in the Neck and Shoulder *Helen James, Janice Brown, Annie Burke-Doe and M. E. Miller*	33
Chapter 4	Neck Pain Induced by Deep Neck Infections *Masahiro Nakayama, Keiji Tabuchi and Akira Hara*	45
Chapter 5	Experimental Neck Muscles Pain, Standing Balance and Proprioception *Nicolas Vuillerme, Petra Hlavackova, Antoine Pradels, Céline Franco and Jacques Vaillant*	57
Chapter 6	Pharmacological Intervention in Management of Neck Pain Disorders: A Review *Marwan S. M. Al-Nimer*	69
Chapter 7	Fear-Avoidance Beliefs-A Challenge to the Traditional Disease Model for Treatment of Neck Pain *Kwok-Chung Lee and Thomas T. W. Chiu*	143
Index		159

PREFACE

Neck pain is often caused by numerous spinal problems including inflammation, muscular tightness in both the neck and upper back, and pinching of the nerves emanating from the cervical vertebrae. Various head and neck lesions such as neck infections can also induce neck pain. In this book, the authors present topical research in the study of neck pain, including the biomechanics, neuroanatomy and neurophysiology of cervical facet joint pain; musculoskeletal discomfort in the neck due to computer use; rolfing structural integration treatment for neck pain; neck pain induced by deep neck infections and pharmacological intervention in the management of neck pain disorders.

Chapter 1 - *Objectives:* The cervical facet joints have been found to be a potentially important source of neck pain or pain referred to the periphery. The authors reviewed the biomechanics, neuroanatomy and neurophysiology of cervical facet joint pain.

Methods: PubMed and MEDLINE databases (1950-2011) were searched for the key words "facet joints," "zygapophyseal joints," and "neck pain." All relevant articles in English were reviewed. Pertinent secondary references were also retrieved.

Results: Clinical studies indicate that the facet joint is the origin of a good percentage of cervical spinal pain. Studies using diagnostic blocks suggest that many of cervical facet joint pain patients have no obvious radiographic abnormalities and pain may be of capsular origin.

Biomechanical studies the support overstretch of cervical facet joint capsules (FJCs) as a possible source of neck pain after whiplash. In particular, axial compression may cause loosing of ligaments and make it easier for the cervical facet joint capsule and other tissues to be injured, while axial head rotation prior to rear impact increases the risk of facet joint injury.

The neuroanatomic and neurophysiologic studies provide the following evidence to help explain the mechanism of cervical facet joint pain: (1) The presence of mechanoreceptive and nociceptive nerve endings demonstrates that cervical facet capsules are monitored by the central nervous system (CNS), and implies that neural input from the facets is important to the function of the cervical spine. (2) Excessive facet capsule stretch, while not producing visible tearing, can produce functional plasticity of dorsal horn neuronal activity. (3) Different joint loading scenarios produced varied inflammatory responses in the CNS. (4) The spinal glutamatergic system may potentiate the persistent behavioral hypersensitivity that is produced following dynamic whiplash-like joint loading. (5) Adolescents may have a lower tissue tolerance to induce pain and associated nociceptive response than do adults. (6)

Associated with the injured facet joints, the phenotypic switch to large neurons may complicate the mechanism of injured facet pain.

Conclusion: An up-to-date knowledge of this subject forms the biomechanical, neuronanatomic and neuronphysiological basis for a hypothesis that the facet joint capsule is a source of neck pain and that the pain may arise from large strain in the joint capsule that will cause pain receptors to fire. However, further studies are needed to validate the clinical application of such hypothesis.

Chapter 2 - Occupational injuries pose a major problem in workplaces where computers are widely used. Intensive, repetitive and long period computer use results in costly health problems (direct cost), and loss of productivity (indirect cost). The causes of musculoskeletal disorders (MSD) in workplaces are diverse and poorly understood. Yet, fewer studies exist on the computer use related musculoskeletal disorders, focusing on musculoskeletal problems in the neck.

In this chapter, the authors will present the findings of a risk assessment model through scientific research to determine the effect of discomfort factors that contribute to musculoskeletal disorders at the neck region resulting from intensive use of computers in workplaces. In this regard a questionnaire was given to 130 intensive computer users working in the university sector. A list of significant predictor variables for musculoskeletal disorders were developed to assess and analyze workplace ergonomics, worker attitudes and experiences due to computer use.

The main focus of the current research is to seek and provide evidence of the symptoms of musculoskeletal discomfort and the frequency of these symptoms which are significant in the development of work-related musculoskeletal disorders (WRMSDs). This study provides the evidence that, ache and pain are the most common types of discomforts in all body regions and the discomforts were pronounced the most in the neck region. The risk factors determined by the risk assessment model were validated through ANOVA of the sEMG records for the control and test groups. The findings indicated that for each test group respondent, although the mean musculoskeletal strain experienced differs in time, the same is not true for the control group.

The potential application of this chapter include the reduction of work-related musculoskeletal disorders associated with the intensive, repetitive and long period computer use that affects the overloaded neck region. Thus, the study provides guidance for solving problems related with costly health problems, lost productivity, and relieve the imposed economic burden.

Chapter 3 - *Background.* Misalignments in the body compromise the architectural integrity. At the tissue level, fascia shortens and thickens as the body engages in compensatory strategies to maintain itself upright, these changes are known as myofascial contractions. Fascia is found all over the body; therefore, when the fascia is altered, the movement capacity is decreased. Dupuytren disease, plantar fibromatosis, club foot, and frozen shoulder are examples of fascial disorders. In physical therapy, there are several methods by which practitioners treat these dysfunctions. However, studies showing the effect of those techniques are limited. *Purpose.* The purpose of studies by Brown (2010) and James, et al (2007) was to investigate the effect of Rolfing Structural Integration (RSI) in either shoulder or neck motion and pain levels of subjects who received RSI from a clinician who was both licensed in physical therapy and had advanced certification in RSI. RSI is a type of therapy that focuses on aligning the human body with gravity. Methods. This retrospective study reported by James et al. over a period of years of clinical practice, analyzes changes in motion and pain levels at the neck for subjects who completed the RSI 10 basic sessions. Participants were evaluated before and after they received RSI. The data collected included: age, sex, occupation, referral source, diagnosis, height, weight, photographs of postural views, range of motion (ROM), pain, and functional complaints. ROM was assessed with the use of an arthordial protractor. Data analysis using three-way ANOVA tested the hypothesis at significance of 0.5. Brown J, (2010) replicated the study using the same clinical data set for the shoulder. Results. The mean *pain* levels and *AROM* before RSI, significantly changed after the treatment ($p < 0.5$), there was a decrease in *pain* and an increase in *AROM*. Pain Levels/AROM-Age within subject effect demonstrated significant difference in *pain at best;* the mean pain levels in the older group decreased by 67%, and the mean AROM for in the younger group increased by 34 %. *Discussion.* In this sample: *Pain now* was reduced more than *pain best* and *pain worst.* Increased motion was reported for groups in both the neck and shoulder studies. *Conclusion.* This investigation demonstrates that the basic 10 sessions of RSI, when applied by a physical therapist with advanced RSI certification, decreases pain and increases AROM in adult subjects male and female with complaints of cervical spine or shoulder dysfunction regardless of age.

Chapter 4 - Neck pain is often caused by numerous spinal problems including inflammation, muscular tightness in both the neck and upper back, and pinching of the nerves emanating from the cervical vertebrae. Various head and neck lesions such as neck infections also induce neck pain. Most deep neck infections were caused by spreading from pharyngeal and odontogenic origins, and induce marked neck pain. Since they may rapidly compromise the airway, and also spread to the mediastinum or cause sepsis, a lack of awareness of these conditions and a delayed diagnosis may lead to potentially fatal consequences. This review discusses the causes, evaluation, and available treatments for the common type of neck pain induced by infections in head and neck regions. Early diagnosis and treatment are essential in order to prevent life-threatening complications.

Chapter 5 - In this study, the authors used an experimental pain model to provide painful stimulation on the neck muscles to assess the effect of neck muscles pain on the control of unperturbed bipedal posture and on neck proprioception. Sixteen young asymptomatic adults voluntarily participated in two separate experiments.

In experiment 1, participants (n=8) were asked to stand upright, as still as possible, in three experimental conditions : (1) a no pain condition, (2) a condition when a painful stimulation was applied to the neck muscles and (3) a condition in which painful stimulation was applied to another body part, the palms of both hands. The centre of foot pressure displacements were recorded using a on a force platform. Results showed that, for the same perceived intensity of the pain, the painful stimulation applied to the neck muscles increased centre of foot pressure displacements, whereas the painful stimulation applied to the palms of both hands did not. Results of experiment 1 demonstrated the deleterious effect of experimentally-induced pain on the neck muscles on unperturbed bipedal postural control and suggest that the painful stimulation affects the postural control mechanisms through sensori-motor mechanisms rather than through cognitive resources related to the perception of pain.

Experiment 2 was specifically designed to address this issue by assessing the effect of on experimental neck muscles pain on cervical joint position sense. To this end, participants (n=8) were asked to execute a clinical test usually employed to the cervical joint position sense, the Cervicocephalic Repositioning Test (CRT) CRT to Neutral Head Position (NHP).

In this assessment, a blindfolded subject seated on a chair with the head in NHP is asked to relocate the head on the trunk, as accurately as possible, after full active cervical rotation to the left and right sides, and absolute and variable errors were used to assess accuracy and consistency of the repositioning, respectively. The CRT to NHP was performed in two experimental conditions presented in Experiment 1: (1) a no pain condition, (2) a condition when a painful stimulation was applied to the neck muscles. Results showed that the painful stimulation applied to the neck muscles induced less accurate and less consistent repositioning performances. Results of experiment 2 demonstrated the deleterious effect of experimentally-induced pain on the neck muscles on cervical joint position sense, assessed through the CRT to the NHP.

Taken together, results of Experiments 1 and 2 suggest experimental neck muscle pain affected control of unperturbed bipedal posture via altered proprioceptive inflow.

Chapter 6 - The prevalence of neck pain disorders is increasing worldwide. Approximately 10% of adult have neck pain at any one time and less than 1% develop neurological deficit. The treatment of neck pain depends on its precise cause. It includes: rest, heat/ice application, traction, soft collar traction, physical therapy, transcutaneous electric nerve stimulation, surgical procedures and pharmacotherapy. The current pharmacological agents that used in management of neck pain include: non steroidal anti-inflammatory drugs, centrally acting analgesia, acetaminophen, muscle relaxants, topical painkillers and/or topical anesthesia, local steroids and/or local anesthetics injections and antimicrobials.

This review focuses on the concepts of pharmacotherapy of neck pain disorders in respect to the cause of neck pain, the nature of pain (acute, chronic, neuropathic or nociceptive), the mechanism of drug action, the practice of local injections with radiologist intervention, quality of life and the long term harmful effects including medicines abused. Also this review describes the beneficial effect of tumor necrosis factor-alpha (TNF-α) blockers, calcitonin gene related peptide antagonists, antimicrobials particularly in infectious cervical discitis and the traditional medicines including natural plants and herbs.

Chapter 7 - Neck pain is a common symptom in the population. Successful management of neck pain is a real challenge to clinicians. Understanding the pain pathways is essential when investigating pain mechanisms and its management. This article gives a brief review of the pain pathways at the simplest form, leading to the fact that pain can be modulated by the past experiences, emotions and cultural background of the person via sensory-discriminative, cognitive-behavioral and affective-emotional mechanisms.

The traditional Cartesian model of specific pain pathways is deeply rooted in the concepts of the clinical management of patients suffering from pain or disease. However, this traditional management for patients with neck pain, from an evidence-based perspective, is now a point of controversy in the literature. On the contrary, a new trend in considering psychosocial factors in the management of spinal pain had been established. There is increasing evidence to support the belief that the clinical presentation of chronic disability could be better understood and managed by using a biopsychosocial model which, as its name implies, considers the influence and interaction of physical, psychological and social factors on human pain perception and behaviors.

Among the psychosocial factors, the fear-avoidance beliefs as set out in the Fear-Avoidance Beliefs Model developed by Lethem et al. have been hypothesized as one of the most important, specific and powerful cognitive variables in predicting disability and treatment outcome in patients with lower back pain. In a recent study involving 120 patients with chronic neck pain the present authors demonstrate that the fear-avoidance belief is an important measure in addition to pain, physical impairments, disability and health status measures. Moreover, the fear-avoidance belief is an important psychosocial factor in predicting the level of future disability and the likelihood of return to complete work capacity at the earlier phase of rehabilitation. These findings lend good support to the recommendation that early identification of patients with high fear-avoidance beliefs would help in planning an appropriate treatment for them to prevent the development of chronic disability and incapacity to work, therefore reducing the socioeconomic impact of neck pain to society.

Neck pain is a common symptom in the population. A review of different observational studies of neck pain over the world showed that the one-year prevalence ranged from 16.7% to 75.1% for the entire adult population (17-70 years) with a mean of 37.2%, and the prevalence is independent of age but higher in women than men (Fejer et al. 2006). Neck pain also causes a significant expense in modern society. The total cost of neck pain in the Netherlands in 1996 was about 1% of the total health care expenditure (Borghouts et al.1999). Neck pain is associated with work absenteeism and restricted work duty in nurses, and its social impact included inadequate sleep as well as reduced participation in non-work activities and recreation (Trinkoff et al. 2002). Therefore, neck pain is a global health problem which greatly affects a person's quality of life. Effective management of patients with neck pain continues to be a real challenge to clinicians.

In: Neck Pain: Causes, Diagnosis and Management
Editor: Gregorio Lombardi

ISBN 978-1-61470-363-1
© 2012 Nova Science Publishers, Inc.

Chapter 1

CERVICAL FACET JOINT PAIN: BIOMECHANICS, NEUROANATOMY AND NEUROPHYSIOLOGY

Haibin Chen[1], Liying Zhang[1,2], Zhengguo Wang[1], John Michael Cavanaugh[2] and King H. Yang[2]

[1]State Key Laboratory of Trauma, Burns, and Combined Injuries, Institute of Surgery Research, Daping Hospital, Third Military Medical University, Chongqing 400042, PR China
[2]Bioengineering Center, Wayne State University, Detroit, Michigan 48202, U. S.

ABSTRACT

Objectives: The cervical facet joints have been found to be a potentially important source of neck pain or pain referred to the periphery. We reviewed the biomechanics, neuroanatomy and neurophysiology of cervical facet joint pain.

Methods: PubMed and MEDLINE databases (1950-2011) were searched for the key words "facet joints," "zygapophyseal joints," and "neck pain." All relevant articles in English were reviewed. Pertinent secondary references were also retrieved.

Results: Clinical studies indicate that the facet joint is the origin of a good percentage of cervical spinal pain. Studies using diagnostic blocks suggest that many of cervical facet joint pain patients have no obvious radiographic abnormalities and pain may be of capsular origin.

Biomechanical studies the support overstretch of cervical facet joint capsules (FJCs) as a possible source of neck pain after whiplash. In particular, axial compression may cause loosing of ligaments and make it easier for the cervical facet joint capsule and other tissues to be injured, while axial head rotation prior to rear impact increases the risk of facet joint injury.

The neuroanatomic and neurophysiologic studies provide the following evidence to help explain the mechanism of cervical facet joint pain: (1) The presence of mechanoreceptive and nociceptive nerve endings demonstrates that cervical facet capsules are monitored by the central nervous system (CNS), and implies that neural input from the facets is important to the function of the cervical spine. (2) Excessive facet capsule stretch, while not producing visible tearing, can produce functional plasticity of dorsal horn neuronal activity. (3) Different joint loading scenarios produced varied inflammatory responses in the CNS. (4) The spinal glutamatergic system may potentiate the persistent behavioral hypersensitivity that is produced following dynamic whiplash-like joint loading. (5) Adolescents may have a lower tissue tolerance to induce pain and associated nociceptive response than do adults. (6) Associated with the injured facet joints, the phenotypic switch to large neurons may complicate the mechanism of injured facet pain.

Conclusion: An up-to-date knowledge of this subject forms the biomechanical, neuronanatomic and neuronphysiological basis for a hypothesis that the facet joint capsule is a source of neck pain and that the pain may arise from large strain in the joint capsule that will cause pain receptors to fire. However, further studies are needed to validate the clinical application of such hypothesis.

INTRODUCTION

The cervical spine facet joint consists of the facet bone, capsular ligament, synovial fluid, synovial membrane and articular cartilage. This complex medium of fluid, hard and soft tissue structures interacts to resist physiologic and traumatic loads, and to maintain strength and stability of the spine.

Morphologically, the cervical joint capsule is well innervated, receiving nerve supply from the medial branches of the dorsal rami, and each medial branch segmentally innervates at two facet joints [1] (Bogduk, 1982).

Facet joints have been found to be a possible source of neck pain or pain referred to the periphery, and a broad range of experiments has been carried out to suggest the mechanism of such cervical spine facet joint pain[2](Chen et al, 2009).

1. CERVICAL FACET JOINT PAIN

Bogduk and Marsland (1988) and Lord et al (1993) maintain that the cervical facet joints are the most common sources of neck pain from whiplash injury [3, 4]. Aprill and Bogduk (1992) reported on a group of 128 patients with chronic neck pain, usually following injury of the whiplash type [5]. These patients had local anesthetic blocks to the nerves innervating the cervical facets and 82 obtained complete relief of their pain. To account for false-positives, a second study was performed on fifty consecutive patients [6](Barnsley et al, 1995). Controlled diagnostic blocks were performed with two types of anesthesia: short-acting lignocaine or longer-acting bupivacaine. Twenty-seven of 38 patients who completed the study had pain relief from both injections and longer duration relief with the bupivacaine. The prevalence of cervical facet pain was concluded to be at least 54% (27 out of 50). A similar study indicated that 55% of patients with chronic, nonspecific cervical spinal pain had pain of facet origin [7](Manchikanti et al, 2004).

A chronic pain condition (late whiplash syndrome) without detectable lesions was also reported to occur in subjects with a whiplash injury of the neck [8, 9] (Borchgrevink et al, 1995; Ronnen et al, 1996). The facet joint is a potential source of pain in these cases.

Percutaneous radiofrequency neurotomy of the dorsal rami branches was shown to offer pain relief by denaturing the nerves that innervate the facet joint at the level of pain [10](Lord et al, 1996). Long-term relief can be maintained by multiple treatments to overcome axon regeneration. Kallakuri et al (2004) demonstrated nerve profiles that were immunoreactive to substance P and calcitonin gene-related peptide in human cervical facet-joint capsules, strongly suggesting that the capsule does contain nerves that can signal pain [11].

Additionally, several studies have linked neck pain and facet joint deformation by studying cervical spine kinematics [12-15](Deng et al, 2000; Kaneoka et al, 1999; Ono et al, 1997; Yoganandan et al, 1998).

Postmortem studies support facet, disc and muscle as possible sources of whiplash pain. Injuries observed included herniations and tears of the intervertebral discs and damage to the facet joints, ligaments and surrounding muscle [16,17](Abel, 1975; Jonsson et al., 1991). Facet joint injury involved tears of the joint capsules hemarthroses and fractures of articular cartilage and subchondral bone [16, 18-20](Buonocore et al, 1966; Wickstrom et al, 1970; Abel, 1975; and Woodring and Goldstein, 1982). A shortcoming of these types of studies is that the severity of impact is typically greater than that of a low-to-moderate speed rear end impact, so the extent of injury is obviously greater.

2. BIOMECHANICS STUDIES

2.1. Axial Compression Hypothesis

In volunteer tests, McConnell et al (1993) found that a vertical acceleration can be measured during a low speed rear-end impact [21]. This ramping up phenomenon was due to the straightening of the spine or the mechanical interaction between the seatback and the torso. This same phenomenon was also reported in a high-speed X-rays study of the neck for volunteers subjected to rear impact forces [22](Matsushita et al, 1994) and in Hybrid II dummy tests by Viano (1992) [23]. However, the measured vertical acceleration and movement were rather small that McConnell et al later reported to be insignificant compared to those measured horizontally [24](McConnell et al, 1995).

Although the vertical acceleration may seem small, it plays a significant role in the cervical spine biomechanics. The head generally possesses about 4.5 kg (10 lbs) of inertial mass. Even a small acceleration could generate a significant compressive force at the neck. In a rear-end impact, the car seat pushes (shears) the torso forward while the neck is subjected to this axial compression. Based on this observation, Yang and Begeman (1996) proposed a new hypothesis to explain the rear-end neck injury mechanism stating that axial compression can cause loosing of ligaments and make it easier for the cervical facet joint capsule and other tissues to be injured [25]. Because these injuries occur in soft tissues, this new theory explains why there is generally no objective evidence.

The facet joint geometry of the cervical spine also plays an important role. In frontal impacts, the upper vertebra will shear anteriorly, relative to the lower vertebra. By observing the anatomy of the facet joints, it is evident that contact of the facet joints can protect against excessive frontal shear. However, in a rear-end impact, the lower vertebra shears anteriorly, the facet joint offers no protection to such a motion. This can be the reason that the rate of neck injury is much lower in frontal impacts of the same or even higher severity.

To test this hypothesis, an in vitro experiment was designed to investigate the theory that axial compression reduces the shear stiffness when the cervical spine is moved due to a rear-end impact [26](Yang and Begeman et al, 1997).

Cervical spine specimens from C1-T1 were dissected from the entire spine. The C1 vertebra was fixed to an aluminum plate with screws. The other end (T1) was potted in epoxy and attached to a six-axis load cell. Two LED markers were attached to each vertebra body from C2-C7. One additional LED maker was attached to the frame of the Instron as reference. During the test, the actuator moves upward to simulate the seat back pushing from behind.

Five tests were done for each specimen. In the first test, the T1 was moved anteriorly to stimulate a rear-end impact for 20 mm (0.79 Inch) displacement at a quasi-static speed of 0.04 mm/s. In the next four tests, an axial compression of 44.5 N (10 lbs), 89.0 N (20 lbs), 133.5 N (30 lbs) and 178 N (40 lbs) of dead weight were applied through a cable-pulley system. The same procedure as in the first test was then reported. Shear stiffness values were calculated from the load cell and motion data.

Result showed that shear stiffness values were reduced significantly with increased axial compression. Based on the total shear force vs the shear deflection data for a typical C5-C6 motion segment, it can be clearly seen that the shear stiffness decreased as the applied axial compression increased. The shear force vs deflection curves were nonlinear due to coupling rotations of vertebrae. The shear stiffness, defined as the final liner portion of the force-deflection curve, reduced significant with increased axial compression. For example, for the C2-C3 portion of the specimen No. 715, the shear stiffness was only 50% of that without axial preload (Table 1).

It should be noted that in previous typical static tests, the shear stiffness is expected to increase as the axial compression increase. Yang (1997)'s experimental data show the opposite trend [26]. This explain why the neck injury rate is higher in a rear-end impact than that of a frontal impact. The axial compression presented in rear-end impact reduce the shear stiffness of the cervical spine and make it easier to be injured. Dynamic tests can give researchers more insight into the neck injury mechanism. Those data can be useful in the design of new equipment such as head restraints to protect the neck from rear-end injury.

Table 1. Shear stiffness values calculated at each vertebra level (Specimen No. 715)

	Stiffness (N/mm)			
	C2-C3	C3-C4	C4-C5	C5-C6
No preload	14.9	9.0	10.9	18.6
178 N preload	7.5	4.5	6.3	5.0

2.2. Axial Pretorque Hypothesis

Whiplash patients who had their head turned at impact have more severe and persistent symptoms than patients who were facing forward [28, 29](Sturzenegger et al, 1994; Sturzenegger et al, 1995). These findings have prompted biomechanical studies using human cadaveric necks to investigate why a head-turned posture increases injury potential. Dynamic rear-impact tests of prerotated ligamentous spines (occiput-T1) produce increased neck flexibility (interpreted as injury) in extension, lateral bending and axial rotation [30](Panjabi et al, 2006). Though concentrated in the lower cervical spine, these "injuries" were not isolated to particular spinal ligaments. Detailed measurements of the strain field in the facet capsule have also shown that a head-turned posture generates higher capsular strains than a neutral head posture, but the quasi-static loads applied during those tests were limited to pure flexion/extension moments and did not include the axial compression or posterior shear present during whiplash loading [31](Winkelstein et al, 2000). Thus the question of how a head-turned posture combined with multiaxial whiplash loads affects facet capsular ligament strain has yet to be answered.

For this reason, Siegmund et al [32](2008) used human cadaveric motion segments to: (1) quantify the intervertebral kinematics and facet capsule strains under whiplash-like loads in the presence of an initial axial rotation, and (2) compare the capsule strains generated by these combined loads to the previously-published strains needed to injure these ligaments in isolated shear failure [33](Siegmund et al, 2001). Their overall hypothesis was that capsular strains during this simulated whiplash exposure are similar to those needed to injure the capsular ligament [32](Siegmund et al, 2008).

According to Siegmund et al (2008), thirteen motion segments were used from 7 women donors (50±10 years). Axial pretorques (±1.5Nm), axial compressive preloads (45, 197, and 325 N), and quasi-static shear loads (posteriorly-directed horizontal forces from 0 to 135 N) were applied to the superior vertebral body to simulate whiplash kinematics with the head turned.

Three-dimensional displacements of markers placed on the right facet capsular ligament were used to estimate the strain field in the ligament during loading. The effects of pretorque direction, compression, and posterior shear on motion segment motion and maximum principal strain in the capsule were examined using repeated-measures analyses of variance.

Results showed that axial pretorque affected peak capsule strains more than axial compression or posterior shear. Peak strains reached 34%±18% and were higher for pretorques toward rather than away from the facet capsule (i.e., head rotation to the right caused higher strain in the right facet capsule).

Similarly, based on a validated intact head to first thoracic vertebra (T1) computational model, parametric analysis was used to assess effects of increasing axial head rotation between 0 and 60°and increasing impact severity between 8 and 24 km/h on facet joint capsule strains [34](Storvik et al, 2011).

Rear impacts were simulated by horizontally accelerating the T1 vertebra. Characteristics of the acceleration pulse were based on the horizontal T1 acceleration pulse from a series of simulated rear impact experiments using full-body post mortem human subjects.

Joint capsule strain magnitudes were greatest in ipsilateral facet joints for all simulations incorporating axial head rotation (i.e., head rotation to the left caused higher ligament strain at the left facet joint capsule). Strain magnitudes increased by 47–196% in simulations with 60° head rotation compared to forward facing simulations. These findings indicate that axial head rotation prior to rear impact increases the risk of facet joint injury.

2.3. Facet Joint Impingement Hypothesis

Ono et al (1997) and Yoganandan et al (1998) both proposed a facet joint impingement hypothesis [14, 15]. Specifically, Ono et al (1997) theorized that the facet synovium or a portion of the facet capsule could be trapped between the facet joint surfaces and pinched, causing pain [14]. However, there is no biomechanical evidence that the capsule is loose enough to be trapped between the facet joint and even if it was trapped, evidence is lacking to show that nociceptors are present in the synovium or the trapped portion of the capsule that is indeed set off by the pressure. Kaneoka et al (1999) hypothesized that the center of rotation moved superiorly during a whiplash and caused the tip of the inferior facet (of the upper vertebra) to impact the superior facet surface (of the lower vertebra) [13]. This proposition that compression of the facet surfaces can produce pain is probably untenable since cartilage is devoid of nociceptors and there is no neurophysiological evidence that the nociceptors in the subchondral bone can be made to fire by this presumed compression.

2.4. Injury Threshold of Cervical Facet Capsule

Biomechanical studies show that facets sustain subfailure strain in whiplash events, strongly suggesting that the facet is a source of pain after whiplash injury. Based on clinical studies Barnley et al (1995) concluded that cervical facet joint pain was the most common source of chronic neck pain after whiplash [6]. Previously, Cavanaugh and colleagues studied the neurophysiology of the lumbar facet joint and published data supporting the facet as a source of low back pain (Cavanaugh, 1996) [27]. More recently, both Cavanaugh and Winkelstein have studied the neurological response to facet capsule stretch in the cervical spine. They and co-workers were able to demonstrate how the facet joint pain can be initiated by overstretch of the facet joint capsule and how that pain can persist. Their studies described below provide a logical physiological background for understanding the mechanisms of facet mediated pain after facet overstretch in rear-end neck injury.

2.4.1. In-Vivo-Goat-Model Based Experiments

An in vivo goat model [35-40](Cavanaugh et al., 2006; Chen et al., 2004, 2005; Lu et al., 2005a, 2005c) was developed to investigate the injury threshold of cervical facet joint capsules (FJC) in vivo. The method incorporated a custom-fabricated testing frame for facet joint loading, a stereoimaging system, and a template-matching technique to obtain single afferent response. The C5 articular process was then pulled via a computer-controlled actuator at a rate of 0.5 mm/sec to simultaneously stretch the C5-6 capsule, record sensory nerve activity due to stretch and record strain by tracking tagets on the capsule. In these studies Lu et al (2005c) demonstrated a quantitative relationship between capsule sensory discharges and applied capsule stretch from cervical facet joints [40]. Neural responses of all mechanosensitive units showed statistically significant correlations (all $P \ll 0.05$) with both capsular load ($r^2 = 0.744 \pm 0.109$) and local strain ($r^2 = 0.868 \pm 0.088$). Most of the capsular neural receptors responded in the physiologic range of capsule stretch and fired at strains of $(10.2 \pm 4.6)\%$ that typically do not signal pain. However, higher capsular strains of $(47.2 \pm 9.6)\%$ triggered discharges from higher threshold receptors which were most likely from nociceptors. Nociceptors transmit signals to the central nervous system to signal pain.

Afterdischarges were reported in these goat studies after capsular strains of (45.0 ± 15.1)% and may be related to tissue injury and release of inflammatory mediators into the surrounding tissue. These changes may lead to central sensitization of pain pathways in the spinal cord which may lead to persistent or chronic whiplash pain. The spinal cord changes that result from facet injury have been investigated by Dr. Winkelstein and the work of her laboratory is described below.

2.4.2. In-Vivo-Rat-Model Based Experiments

Quinn et al (2007) conducted a study to quantify the structural mechanics of the cervical facet capsule and define the threshold for altered structural responses in this ligament during distraction [41].

Tensile failure tests were performed using isolated C6/C7 rat facet capsular ligaments (n = 8); gross ligament failure, the occurrence of minor ruptures and ligament yield were measured. Gross failure occurred at (2.45 ± 0.60)N and (0.92 ± 0.17)mm. However, the yield point occurred at (1.68 ± 0.56)N and (0.57 ± 0.08)mm, which was significantly less than gross failure (p<0.001 for both measurements). Maximum principal strain in the capsule at yield was (80 ± 24)%. Energy to yield was (14.3 ± 3.4)% of the total energy for a complete tear of the ligament. Ligament yield point occurred at a distraction magnitude in which pain symptoms begin to appear in vivo in the rat.

Findings presented here suggest a relationship between structural damage of the facet capsular ligament and potential mechanisms of pain for subfailure distraction. Quinn et al (2007)'s data show ligament yield at a significantly lower distraction than gross failure [41]. While these subfailure distractions may not produce visible ligament tears, detection of the ligament's altered structural response may provide an indication of an injury sufficient to elicit sustained nociceptor firing, pain symptoms, and persistent activity in the nervous system.

Given the evidence that painful joint distractions begin near ligament yield, this study may suggest that the physiologic range of the facet joint is actually limited to prior to yield. This mechanical study provides a framework for future in vivo studies in determining a mechanical threshold for persistent pain, and also provides data for quantitative scaling to other animal models and to the human. These findings provide mechanical definition of altered ligament behavior corresponding with a loading condition known to produce pain, linking mechanical damage and persistent pain for the first time.

3. NEUROANATOMIC STUDIES

For facets to be a source of pain after whiplash, the facet joint capsule must contain nerve endings, including nerve endings that signal pain. To help address issue, Mclain et al (1993) [42] examined normal cervical facet capsules, taken from three human subjects, to determine the density and distribution of three types of mechanoreceptive nerve endings in Mclain (1993)'s studies. Clearly identifiable mechanoreceptors were found in 80% of the specimens and were categorized according to the classification of Freeman and Wyke [43]. Eleven Type I, twenty Type II, and five Type III receptors were identified, as well as a number of small, unencapsulated nerve endings (Table 2).

Table 2. Classification of Nerve Endings According to Freeman and Wyke (1967)

TYPE	MORPHOLOGY	PARENT NERVES	FUNCTION
I	Globular corpuscles in clusters. Thinly encapsulated.	Small myelinated fibers.	Static, dynamic; low threshold, slowly adapting.
II	Conical corpuscles, thickly encapsulated.	Medium myelinated fibers.	Dynamic receptors; low threshold, rapidly adapting.
III	Fusiform corpuscles, thinly encapsulated.	Large myelinated fibers.	Dynamic receptors; high threshold, very slowly adapting.
IV	Free nerve endings.	Very small myelinated. Unmyelinated.	Pain receptors; high threshold, non-adapting.

Type I receptors were small, globular structures measuring 25-50 microns in diameter. Type II receptors varied in size and contour, but were characterized by their oblong shape and broad, lamellar capsule. Type III receptors were relatively large, oblong structures with a thin, amorphous capsule, within which a reticular mesh-work of fine neurites was embedded. Free (nociceptive) nerve endings were found in sub-synovial, loose areolar, and dense capsular tissues. Fine, unmyelinated nerves consistent with Type IV receptors (less than five microns) were identified in both the dense capsular tissues and in the synovial and areolar tissues; these fine filaments most likely represent nociceptive nerve endings. Such fibers also accompanied many of the vessels within the dense fibrous tissue of the capsule.

The presence of mechanoreceptive and nociceptive nerve endings demonstrates that cervical facet capsules are monitored by the central nervous system, and implies that neural input from the facets is important to the function of the cervical spine. Previous study [11] has suggested that protective muscular reflexes modulated by these types of mechanoreceptors are important in preventing joint instability and degeneration.

4. NEUROPHYSIOPATHOLOGICAL STUDIES

4.1. Axonal Changes in Stretched Cervical Facet Joint Capsule

Kallakuri et al (2008)'s study examines axonal changes in goat cervical facet joint capsules (FJC) subjected to low rate loading [44]. Left C5–C6 FJC was subjected to a series of tensile tests from 2 mm to failure using a computer-controlled actuator. The FJC strain on the dorsal aspect was monitored by a stereo-imaging system. Stretched (n = 10) and unstretched (n = 7) capsules were harvested and serial sections were processed by a silver impregnation method. The mean peak actuator displacement was 21.3 mm (range: 12–30 mm). The average peak strain encompassing various regions of the capsule was (72.9 ± 7.1)%. Complete failure of the capsule was observed in 70% of the stretched capsules. Silver impregnation of the sections revealed nerve fibers and bundles in all the regions of the capsule. A blinded analysis of digital photomicrographs of axons revealed a statistically significant number of swollen axons with non-uniform caliber in stretched FJCs. Axons with terminal retraction balls, with occasional beaded appearance or with vacuolations were also observed. Stretching the FJC beyond physiological range could result in altered axonal morphology that may be related to secondary or delayed axotomy changes similar to those seen in central nervous system injuries where axons are subjected to stretching and shearing. These may contribute to neuropathic pain and are potentially related to neck pain after whiplash events.

4.2. Infammatory Responses and Pain Symptoms from Cervical Facet Joint

According to Lee et al [45](2008), two joint loading paradigms were used separately in an established rat model [46](Lee et al, 2004) of painful cervical facet joint distraction to apply: (1) gross failure, and (2) subfailure distraction of the facet capsular ligament. Behavioral outcomes were compared to determine whether more severe mechanical loading produces greater pain by measuring mechanical hyperalgesia in the shoulder and forepaws. Inflammatory mediators (glia and cytokines) were quantified in the spinal cord and dorsal root ganglion (DRG) after injury. Subfailure loading produced sustained hyperalgesia in the shoulder and forepaw that was significantly greater ($p < 0.042$) than sham, while an induced capsule failure produced only transient, yet significant ($p < 0.021$), mechanical hyperalgesia. The absence of hyperalgesia after ligament failure suggests this type of injury may interrupt nociceptive input from the capsule, which is likely necessary to produce sustained pain symptoms. Glial mRNA was significantly increased ($p < 0.043$) in the spinal cord after ligament failure, but remained unchanged in the DRG. Cytokine mRNA levels in the spinal cord and DRG were also significantly elevated after facet ligament failure, but not after painful subfailure loading. Findings suggest that different joint loading scenarios produced varied inflammatory responses in the central nervous system (CNS). These data support existing clinical reports suggesting that therapeutic interventions directed at the facet capsule may be effective in treating this painful injury.

4.3. Spinal Glutamatergic Response in Cervical Facet Joint Pain

Both the metabotropic glutamate receptor 5 (mGluR5) and the excitatory amino acid carrier 1 (EAAC1) have pivotal roles in chronic pain. According to Dong and Winkelstein (2010), spinal mGluR5 and EAAC1 were quantified following painful facet joint distraction in a rat model of facet-mediated painful loading and were evaluated for their correlation with the severity of capsule loading [47]. Rats underwent either a dynamic C6-C7 joint distraction simulating loading experienced during whiplash (distraction; n = 12) or no distraction (sham; n = 6) to serve as control. The severity of capsular loading was quantified using strain metrics, and mechanical allodynia was assessed after surgery. Spinal cord tissue was harvested at day 7 and the expression of mGluR5 and EAAC1 were quantified using Western blot analysis. Mechanical allodynia following distraction was significantly ($p < 0.001$) higher than sham. Spinal expression of mGluR5 was also significantly ($p < 0.05$) greater following distraction relative to sham. However, spinal EAAC1 was significantly ($p = 0.0003$) reduced compared to sham. Further, spinal mGluR5 expression was significantly positively correlated to capsule strain (p < 0.02) and mechanical allodynia (p < 0.02). Spinal EAAC1 expression was significantly negatively related to one of the strain metrics (p < 0.003) and mechanical allodynia at day 7 (p = 0.03). These results suggest that the spinal glutamatergic system may potentiate the persistent behavioral hypersensitivity that is produced following dynamic whiplash-like joint loading; chronic whiplash pain may be alleviated by blocking mGluR5 expression and/or enhancing glutamate transport through the neuronal transporter EAAC1.

4.4. Age-Related Cervical Facet Joint Pain

There is growing evidence that neck pain is common in adolescence and is a risk factor for the development of chronic neck pain in adulthood. Weisshaar et al (2010) conducted a study to define the biomechanics, behavioral sensitivity, and indicators of neuronal and glial activation in an adolescent model of mechanical facet joint injury [48]. A bilateral C6–C7 facet joint distraction was imposed in an adolescent rat and biomechanical metrics were measured during injury. Following injury, forepaw mechanical hyperalgesia was measured, and protein kinase C-epsilon (PKCe) and metabotropic glutamate receptor-5 (mGluR5) expression in the dorsal root ganglion and markers of spinal glial activation were assessed. Joint distraction induced significant mechanical hyperalgesia during the 7 days post-injury (p < 0.001). Painful injury significantly increased PKCe expression in small- and medium-diameter neurons compared to sham (p < 0.05) and naive tissue (p < 0.001). Similarly, mGluR5 expression was significantly elevated in small-diameter neurons after injury (p < 0.05). Spinal astrocytic activation after injury was also elevated over sham (p < 0.035) and naive (p < 0.0001) levels; microglial activation was only greater than naive levels (p < 0.006). Mean strains in the facet capsule during injury were (32.8 ± 12.9)%, which were consistent with the strains associated with comparable degrees of hypersensitivity in the adult rat. These results suggest that adolescents may have a lower tissue tolerance to induce pain and associated nociceptive response than do adults.

4.5. Neuronal Hyperexcitablility after Cervical Facet Joint Loading

In Quinn et al (2010)'s experiments, using a rat model of C6–C7 cervical facet joint capsule stretch that produces sustained mechanical hyperalgesia, the presence of neuronal hyperexcitability was characterized 7 days after joint loading [49]. Extracellular recordings of spinal dorsal horn neuronal activity between C6 and C8 (117 neurons) were obtained from anesthetized rats, with both painful and non-painful behavioral outcomes established by the magnitude of capsule stretch. The frequency of neuronal firing during noxious pinch (p < 0.0182) and von Frey filaments applications (4–26 g) to the forepaw was increased (p < 0.0156) in the painful group compared to the non-painful and sham groups. In addition, the incidence and frequency of spontaneous and after discharge firing were greater in the painful group (p < 0.0307) relative to sham. The proportion of cells in the deep laminae that responded as wide dynamic range neurons also was increased in the painful group relative to non-painful or sham groups (p < 0.0348). These findings suggest that excessive facet capsule stretch, while not producing visible tearing, can produce functional plasticity of dorsal horn neuronal activity. The increase in neuronal firing across a range of stimulus magnitudes observed at day 7 post-injury provides the first direct evidence of neuronal modulation in the spinal cord following facet joint loading, and suggests that facet-mediated chronic pain following whiplash injury is driven, at least in part, by central sensitization.

4.6. Pathoplysiology of the Intensity and Expansion of Cervical Facet Joint Pain

Ohtori et al (2003) carried out a pathophysiologic investigation of the intensity and expansion of cervical facet joint pain [50]. Retrograde transport of fluoro-gold (F-G) and immunohistochemistry of calcitonin gene-related peptide (CGRP) was used in 20 rats (control group, $n=10$; injured group, $n=10$). For the injured group, the whole facet capsule was incised. Of the total F-G labelled dorsal root ganglion (DRG) neurons innervating the C5/6 facet joint, the number and the cross-sectional area of cell profiles of F-G labelled CGRP-ir neurons were evaluated in the bilateral DRGs of both groups. The numbers of CGRP-ir F-G labelled DRG neurons as a percentage of all F-G labelled DRG neurons at C3, C4, C5, C6, C7, C8, T1, T2, and T3 respectively were 30, 22, 43, 47, 21, 19, 25, 36 and 30% in the control group, and 13, 15, 23, 17, 15, 8, 16, 28 and 35% in the injured group, with the injured group showing a significantly lower percentage of CGRP-ir F-G labelled neurons than the control group at C5 and C6 ($P < 0.05$). However, the mean cross-sectional area of F-G labelled CGRP-ir cells from C3 to C8 DRGs increased from (625 ± 22) μm^2 to (878 ± 33) μm^2 in the injured group ($P < 0.001$). Associated with the injured facet joints, the phenotypic switch to large neurons may complicate the mechanism of injured facet pain.

CONCLUSION

Clinical studies indicate that the facet joint is the origin of a good percentage of cervical spinal pain. Studies using diagnostic blocks suggest that many of cervical facet joint pain patients have no obvious radiographic abnormalities and pain may be of capsular origin.

Biomechanical studies support overstretch of cervical facet joint capsules (FJCs) as a possible source of neck pain after whiplash events. In particular, axial compression may cause loosing of ligaments and make it easier for the cervical facet joint capsule and other tissues to be injured, while axial head rotation prior to rear impact increases the risk of facet joint injury.

The neuroanatomic and neurophysiologic studies provide the following evidence to help explain the mechanism of cervical facet joint pain: (1) The presence of mechanoreceptive and nociceptive nerve endings demonstrates that cervical facet capsules are monitored by the central nervous system (CNS), and implies that neural input from the facets is important to the function of the cervical spine. (2) Excessive facet capsule stretch, while not producing visible tearing, can produce functional plasticity of dorsal horn neuronal activity. (3) Different joint loading scenarios produced varied inflammatory responses in the CNS. (4) The spinal glutamatergic system may potentiate the persistent behavioral hypersensitivity that is produced following dynamic whiplash-like joint loading. (5) Adolescents may have a lower tissue tolerance to induce pain and associated nociceptive response than do adults. (6)

Associated with the injured facet joints, the phenotypic switch to large neurons may complicate the mechanism of injured facet pain.

An up-to-date knowledge of this subject forms the biomechanical, neuronanatomic and neuronphysiological basis for a hypothesis that the facet joint capsule is a source of neck pain and that the pain may arise from large strain in the joint capsule that will cause pain receptors to fire. However, further studies are needed to validate the clinical application of such hypothesis.

ACKNOWLEDGMENTS

This work was supported by grants from the National Natural Science Foundation of China (No. 30928005), the Chongqing Natural Science Foundation of China (No. CSTC2009BB5013), and the Third Military Medical University Research Foundation of China (No. 2009XHG16).

REFERENCES

[1] Bogduk, N. The clinical anatomy of the cervical doral rami. *Spine*, 1982; 7, 319-330.
[2] Chen, HB; Yang, KH; Wang, ZG. Biomechanics of whiplash injury. *Chin. J. Traumatol.*, 2009; 12(5), 305-314.
[3] Bogduk, N; Marsland, A. The cervical zygapophysial joints as a source of neck pain. *Spine*, 1988; 13(6), 610-617.
[4] Lord, S; Barnsley, L; Bogduk, N. Cervical zygapophyseal joint pain in whiplash. In: Spine: Cervical Flexion-Extension/*Whiplash Injuries*, 1993; 7(3), 355-372.
[5] Aprill, C; and Bogduk, N. The prevalence of cervical zygapophyseal joint pain: a first approximation. *Spine*, 1992; 17, 744-747.
[6] Barnsley, L; Lord, S; Wallis, BJ; Bogduk, N. The presence of cervical zygapophyseal joint pain after whiplash. *Spine*, 1995; 20(1), 20-26.
[7] Manchikanti, L; Boswell, MV; Singh, V; Pampati, V; Damron, KS; Beyer, CD. Prevalence of facet joint pain in chronic spinal pain of cervical, thoracic, and lumbar regions. *BMC Musculoskelet Disord*, 2004; 5, 15.
[8] Borchgrevink, GE; Smevik, O; Nordby, A; Rinck, PA; Stiles, TC; Lereim, I. MR imaging and radiography of patients with cervical hypertension-flexion injuries after car accidents. *Acta Radiol*, 1995; 36, 425-8.
[9] Ronnen, HR; de Korte, PJ; Brink, PR; van der Bijl, HJ; Tonino, AJ; Franke, CL. Acute whiplash injury: is there a role for MR imaging?---a prospective study of 100 patients. *Radiology*, 1996; 201, 93-6.
[10] Lord, SM; Barnsley, L; Wallis, BJ; McDonald, GJ; Bogduk, N. Percutaneous radiofrequency neurotomy for chronic cervical zygapophyseal-joint pain. *N. Engl. J. Med.*, 1996; 335, 1721-6.
[11] Kallakuri, S; Singh, A; Chen, C; Cavanaugh, JM. Demonstration of substance P, calcitonin gene-related peptide, and protein gene product 9.5 containing nerve fibers in human cervical facet joint capsules. *Spine*, 2004; 29, 1182-6.

[12] Deng, B; Begeman, PC; Yang, KH; Tashman, S; King, AL. Kinematics of human cadaver cervical spine during low speed reatend impacts. *J. Stapp. Assoc Paper no*, 2000-01-SC13.

[13] Kaneoka, K; Ono, K; Inami, S; Hayashi, K. Motion analysis of cervical vertebrae during whiplash loading. *Spine*, 1999; 24(8), 763-770.

[14] Ono, K; Kaneoka, K; Wittek, A; Kajzer, J. Cervical injury mechanism based on the analysis of human cervical vertebral motion and head-neck-torso kinematics during low speed rear impacts. *Proc. 41st Stapp Car Crash Conference,* Warrendale, PA, Society of Automotive Engineers, 973340, 1997; 339-356.

[15] Yoganandan, N; Pintar, FA; Klienberger M. Cervical spine vertebral and facet joint kinematics under whiplash. *J. Biomech. Eng*. 1998; 120(2), 305-7.

[16] Abel, MS. Occult traumatic lesions of the cervical vertebrae. *Crit. Rev. Clin. Radiol. and Nucl. Med*, 1975; 6, 469-553.

[17] Jonsson, H; Bring, G; Rauschning, W; Sahlstedt, B. Hidden cervical spine injuries in traffic accident victims with skull fractures. *J. Spinal. Disord*, 1991; 4, 251-23.

[18] Buonocore, E; Hartman, JT; and Nelson, CL. Cineradiograms of cervical spine in diagnosis of soft-tissue injuries. *JAMA*, 1966; 198, 143-147.

[19] Wickstrom, J; Martinez, JL; Rodriguez, R; Jr and Haines, DM. Hyperextension and hyperflexion injuries to the head and neck of primates. In: Gurdjian ES, Thomas LM, eds. *Neckache and Backache*. IL: Springfield; 1970; 108-19.

[20] Woodring, JH and Goldstein, SJ. Fractures of the articular processes of the cervical spine. *AJR Am. J. Roentgenol.*, 1982; 139, 341-44.

[21] McConnell, WE; Howard, RP; Guzman, HM; Bomar, JB; Raddin, JH; Benedict, JV; Smith, HL. *Analysis of human test subject kinematic responses to low velocity rear end impacts*. Society for Automobile Engineers, 1993; 21–30.

[22] Matsushita T, Sato TB, Hirabayashi K, Fujimura S, Asaszuma. X-ray study of the human neck motion due to head inertial loading.. *Proc. 39th Stapp Car Crash Conf,* SAE Paper No 942208, 1994; 55-64.

[23] Viano, DC. Influence of seatback angle on occupant dynamics in stimulated rear-end impacts. *SAE*, 1992; 922521.

[24] McConnell, WE; Howard, RP; Van, PJ; Krause, R; Guzman, HM; Bomar, JB; Raddin, JH; Benedict, JV; Hatsell, CP. Human head and neck kinematics after low velocity rear-end impacts-understanding 'whiplash'. *Proc. 39th Stapp Car Crash Conf,* SAE, 1995; 215-238.

[25] Yang, KH; Begman, PC. A proposed role for facet joints in neck pain in low to moderate speed rear end impacts. Part I: Biomechanics. In: 6th Injury Prevention Through Biomechanics Symposium, *WSU,* 1996, 59-63.

[26] Yang, KH; Begeman, PC; Muuser, M; Niederer P, Walz, F. On the Role of Cervical Facet Joints in Rear End Impact Neck Injury Mechanisms. *SAE,* Paper No,970497,1997.

[27] Cavanaugh, JM. A proposed role for facet joints in neck pain in low to moderate speed rear end impacts. *Part II: neuroanatomy and neurophysiology 6th injury prevention through biomechanics symposium*, 1996; 65-71.

[28] Sturzenegger, M; DiStefano, G; Radanov, BP. Presenting symptoms and signs after whiplash injury: the influence of accident mechanisms. *Neurology*, 1994; 44, 688–93.

[29] Sturzenegger, M; Radanov, BP; Di Stefano, G. The effect of accident mechanisms and initial findings on the long-term course of whiplash injury. *J. Neurol*, 1995; 242, 443-9.
[30] Panjabi, MM; Ivancic, PC; Maak, TG. Multiplanar cervical spine injury due to head-turned rear impact. *Spine*, 2006; 31,420-9.
[31] Winkelstein, BA; Nightingale, RW; Richardson, WJ. The cervical facet capsule and its role in whiplash injury: a biomechanical investigation. *Spine*, 2000; 25, 1238-46.
[32] Siegmund, GP; Davis, MB; Quinn, KP; Hines, E; Myers, BS; Ejima, S; Ono, K; Kamiji, K; Yasuki, T; Winkelstein, BA. Head-turned postures increase the risk of cervical facet capsule injury during whiplash. *Spine*, 2008; 33(15), 1643-9.
[33] Siegmund GP, Myers BS, Davis MB, et al. Mechanical evidence of cervical facet capsule injury during whiplash: a cadaveric study using combined shear, compression, and extension loading. *Spine*, 2001; 26, 2095-101.
[34] Storvik, SG; Stemper, BD. Axial head rotation increases facet joint capsular ligament strains in automotive rear impact. *Med. Biol. Eng. Comput*, 2011; 49(2), 153-61.
[35] Cavanaugh, JM; Lu, Y; Chen, C; Kallakuri, S. Pain generation in lumbar and cervical facet joints. *J. Bone Joint Surg. Am.*, 2006; 88 Suppl 2, 63-7.
[36] Chen, C; Lu, Y; Cavanaugh, JM; Kallakuri, S; Patwardhan, A. Neurophysiologic studies of cervical facet joint capsule—experimental setup and characterization of sensory receptors. In: *Transactions of the ORS 50th annual meeting*. 2004.
[37] Chen, C; Lu, Y; Cavanaugh, JM; Kallakuri, S; Patwardhan, A. Recording of neural activity from goat cervical facet joint capsule using custom-designed miniature electrodes. *Spine*, 2005; 30, 1367-72.
[38] Lu, Y; Chen, C; Kallakuri, S; Patwardhan, A; Cavanaugh, JM. Development of an in vivo method to investigate biomechanical and neurophysiological properties of spine facet joint capsules. *Eur. Spine J.*, 2005a; 14(6), 565-72.
[39] Lu,Y; Chen, C; Kallakuri, S; Patwardhan, A; Cavanaugh, JM. Neural response of cervical facet joint capsule to stretch: a study of whiplash pain mechanism. *Stapp Car Crash Journal*, 2005b; 49, 49-56.
[40] Lu, Y; Chen, C; Kallakuri, S; Patwardhan, A; Cavanaugh, JM. Neurophysiological and biomechanical characterization of goat cervical facet joint capsules. *J. Orthop Res.*, 2005c; 23, 779-87.
[41] Quinn, KP; Winkelstein, BA. Cervical facet capsular ligament yield defines the threshold for injury and persistent joint-mediated neck pain. *J. Biomech*, 2007; 40(10), 2299-306.
[42] McLain, RF. Mechanoreceptor endings in human cervical facet joints. *Iowa Orthop J.*, 1993; 13, 149-54.
[43] Freeman, MA; Wyke, BD. The innervation of the knee joint: an anatomical and histological study in the cat. *J. Anat*, 1967; 101, 505-532.
[44] Kallakuri, S; Singh, A; Lu, Y; Chen, C; Patwardhan, A; Cavanaugh, JM. Tensile stretching of cervical facet joint capsule and related axonal changes. *Eur. Spine J.*, 2008; 17(4), 556-63.
[45] Lee, KE; Davis, MB; Winkelstein, BA. Capsular ligament involvement in the development of mechanical hyperalgesia after facet joint loading: behavioral and inflammatory outcomes in a rodent model of pain. *J. Neurotrauma*, 2008; 25(11), 1383-93.

[46] Lee, KE; Davis, MB; Mejilla, RM; Winkelstein, BA. In vivo cervical facet capsule distraction: mechanical implications for whiplash and neck pain. *Stapp Car. Crash J.,* 2004; 48, 373-95.

[47] Dong, L; Winkelstein, BA. Simulated whiplash modulates expression of the glutamatergic system in the spinal cord suggesting spinal plasticity is associated with painful dynamic cervical facet loading. *J. Neurotrauma*, 2010; 27(1), 163-74.

[48] Weisshaar, CL; Dong, L; Bowman, AS; Perez, FM; Guarino, BB; Sweitzer, SM; Winkelstein, BA. Metabotropic glutamate receptor-5 and protein kinase C-epsilon increase in dorsal root ganglion neurons and spinal glial activation in an adolescent rat model of painful neck injury. *J. Neurotrauma,* 2010; 27(12), 2261-71.

[49] Quinn, KP; Dong, L; Golder, FJ; Winkelstein, BA. Neuronal hyperexcitability in the dorsal horn after painful facet joint injury. *Pain.* 2010; 151(2), 414-21.

[50] Ohtori, S; Takahashi, K; Moriya, H. Calcitonin gene-related peptide immunoreactive DRG neurons innervating the cervical facet joints show phenotypic switch in cervical facet injury in rats. *Eur. Spine J.,* 2003; 12(2), 211-5.

In: Neck Pain: Causes, Diagnosis and Management
Editor: Gregorio Lombardi

ISBN 978-1-61470-363-1
© 2012 Nova Science Publishers, Inc.

Chapter 2

WORK-RELATED MUSCULOSKELETAL DISCOMFORT IN THE NECK DUE TO COMPUTER USE

Orhan Korhan[*]
Department of Industrial Engineering
Eastern Mediterranean University
Gazimağusa, North Cyprus
Mersin 10, Turkey

ABSTRACT

Occupational injuries pose a major problem in workplaces where computers are widely used. Intensive, repetitive and long period computer use results in costly health problems (direct cost), and loss of productivity (indirect cost). The causes of musculoskeletal disorders (MSD) in workplaces are diverse and poorly understood. Yet, fewer studies exist on the computer use related musculoskeletal disorders, focusing on musculoskeletal problems in the neck.

In this chapter we will present the findings of a risk assessment model through scientific research to determine the effect of discomfort factors that contribute to musculoskeletal disorders at the neck region resulting from intensive use of computers in workplaces. In this regard a questionnaire was given to 130 intensive computer users working in the university sector. A list of significant predictor variables for musculoskeletal disorders were developed to assess and analyze workplace ergonomics, worker attitudes and experiences due to computer use.

The main focus of the current research is to seek and provide evidence of the symptoms of musculoskeletal discomfort and the frequency of these symptoms which are significant in the development of work-related musculoskeletal disorders (WRMSDs). This study provides the evidence that, ache and pain are the most common types of discomforts in all body regions and the discomforts were pronounced the most in the neck region. The risk factors determined by the risk assessment model were validated through ANOVA of the sEMG records for the control and test groups. The findings

---

[*] Asst. Prof. Dr. Orhan Korhan. Department of Industrial Engineering, Eastern Mediterranean University, Famagusta, TRNC, Mersin 10 TURKEY, Email: orhan.korhan@emu.edu.tr Tel: +90 392 630 1052

indicated that for each test group respondent, although the mean musculoskeletal strain experienced differs in time, the same is not true for the control group.

The potential application of this chapter include the reduction of work-related musculoskeletal disorders associated with the intensive, repetitive and long period computer use that affects the overloaded neck region. Thus the study provides guidance for solving problems related with costly health problems, lost productivity, and relieve the imposed economic burden.

1. INTRODUCTION

The National Institute for Occupational Safety and Health (NIOSH) in the USA defines a Musculoskeletal Disorder (MSD) as a disorder that affects a part of the body's musculoskeletal system, which includes bones, nerves, tendons, ligaments, joints, cartilage, blood vessels and spinal discs. These are the injuries that result from repeated motions, vibrations and forces placed on human bodies while performing various job actions. The factors that can contribute to musculoskeletal symptoms include heredity, physical condition, previous injury, pregnancy, poor diet, and lifestyle.

Work-related musculoskeletal symptoms occur when there is a mismatch between the physical requirements of the job and the physical capacity of the human body. Musculoskeletal disorders are work-related when the work activities and work conditions significantly contribute to their development, but not necessarily the sole or significant determinant of causation.

Work-related musculoskeletal disorders (WRMSDs) describe a wide range of inflammatory and degenerative conditions affecting the muscles, tendons, ligaments, joint, peripheral nerves, and supporting blood vessels. These conditions result in pain and functional impairment and may affect especially the neck.

The causes of musculoskeletal disorders in the workplace are diverse and poorly understood. The meaning that working has to an individual may help to explain why certain psychological factors are associated with musculoskeletal discomfort and may eventually provide one way to intervene to reduce MSD.

Musculoskeletal disorders have been observed and experienced widely at workplaces where the computers are frequently used. Increase in the number of employees working with computer and mouse coincides with an increase of work-related musculoskeletal disorders (WRMSDs) and sick leave, which affects the physical health of workers and pose financial burdens on the companies, governmental and non-governmental organizations.

This chapter presents the factors that contribute to musculoskeletal disorders resulting from intensive use of computers in the workplaces.

The risk factors of musculoskeletal disorders were revealed by assessing and analyzing workplace ergonomics, worker attitudes and experiences on the use of the computer keyboard and mouse. This was followed by an experimental data collection of muscle load, muscle force and muscular fatigue by Surface electromyogram (sEMG) to validate and verify the developed mathematical model.

2. METHODOLOGY

2.1. Objectives

This research addresses worker perception and attitudes towards computer use, and their experiences with musculoskeletal symptoms in the neck and their diagnoses. The primary aim of this chapter is to present an in-debt assessment of the association between work-related musculoskeletal disorders in the neck and computer use.

This study illustrates the idea of understanding how demographic structure, physical and psychosocial job characteristics, office ergonomics, perceived musculoskeletal discomfort types and their frequencies may affect formation of musculoskeletal disorders in the neck. It then provides the evidence on the symptoms of musculoskeletal discomfort types and the frequency of these discomforts which are significant in the development of WRMSD in the neck due to computer use.

The relevance of this study to the industry is to reduce the work-related musculoskeletal disorders associated with the intensive, repetitive and long period computer use that affect the neck. The developed risk assessment model also provides guidance for solving problems related with costly health problems (direct cost), lost productivity (indirect cost), and relieve the imposed economic burden.

As a summary, the research objectives of this study are:

- To assess and to analyze workplace ergonomics, worker attitudes and experiences on computer use, and musculoskeletal symptoms in the neck developed by computer use,
- To determine a meaningful and statistically significant relationship exists between work-related musculoskeletal disorders in the neck and computer use, and develop a risk assessment model,
- To validate and verify the developed mathematical model through analysis of the data collected by the SEMG recordings.

2.2. Questionnaire

A questionnaire was developed based on the U.S. *National Institute for Occupational Safety and Health* (NIOSH) Symptoms Survey and the Nordic Musculoskeletal Questionnaire. The questionnaire included questions in 7 modules according to the type of the questions.

The questions were related with the demographic structure of the participant, physical job characteristics, psychosocial job characteristics, office ergonomics (workstation setup), types of musculoskeletal discomforts experienced at the neck, frequency of the musculoskeletal discomforts in the neck, and personal medical history.

2.3. Experimentation

The respondents of the questionnaire, who have experienced musculoskeletal symptoms, were invited to a lab experiment, where surface electromyogram (sEMG) was used to record muscle load, muscle force and muscular fatigue. This test was taken place in two phases;

- interrupting the work and performing test contractions of known force in a predetermined body posture and,
- comparing situations connected with a certain reference activity.

Before conducting the sEMG experiment, those respondents who were under high risk of having WRMSD in the neck were identified using logistic regression. The significance level in logistic regression analysis was chosen to be 5% in order to minimize the possibility of making a Type I error. An independent variable with a regression coefficient not significantly different from 0 ($p>0.05$) can be removed from the regression model. If $p<0.05$ then the variable contributes significantly to the prediction of the outcome variable (Pampel, 2000).

Odd ratios of the significant factors for each respondent were calculated to find out respondents who were at the risk of having WRMSD in the neck, as given below:

If χ_i's ($i=1,2,\ldots$) are independent variables, then the odds ratio is defined as

$$\log\left[\frac{\text{Prob}(\text{diagnosis of WRMSD})}{\text{Prob}(\text{NOT diagnosis of WRMSD})}\right] = \beta_0 + \beta_1\chi_1 + \beta_2\chi_2 + \ldots$$

where β_0 is the intercept, and $\beta_1, \beta_2, \ldots$ are the regression coefficients.

Thus, we have

$$\text{Odds Ratio} = e^{(\beta_0 + \beta_1\chi_1 + \beta_2\chi_2 + \ldots)}$$

In order to determine the respondents under high risk of having WRMSD in the neck, the odds ratios of the significant factors for each respondent were calculated and those respondents who reflect maximum levels of odds ratios for each significant factor were invited for further investigation through electromyography.

Surface electromyogram was used to collect data from the neck. The procedure for the experimentation was as follows; twenty minutes typing exercise was given to each respondent at a time.

Data were collected at 5th, 10th, 15th, and 20th minutes of the experiment. The mean value of the data collected for 30 seconds was then calculated and taken into consideration. Analysis of Variance (ANOVA) and Factorial Analysis were applied at the end to the data collected by sEMG recordings, to validate and verify the significant risk factors of WRMSD in the neck which were determined by logistic regression.

2.4. Respondents

A questionnaire was given to 130 persons, who worked intensively with the computers for work/business purposes, such as; staff, research assistants and faculty members of Eastern Mediterranean University (EMU), web page designers, computer programmers, engineers, government officers, public relation officers, marketing officers, bank officers, customer representatives, commissioners, consultants, travel agents and translators. The reason for targeting such diverse disciplines is that the target population is expected to use computers intensively especially for work/business purposes and several other auxiliary purposes including personal and communication. Thus the results are guaranteed not to be task-related, instead work-related.

3. RESULTS

3.1. Descriptive Statistics

Seventy male respondents (53.85%) attended this research. The males appeared to be dominating the female respondents (60, 46.15%). Figure 1 illustrates that 107 (82.31%) of the 130 participants were between 20 to 35 years old.

The majority of the respondents (30.77%) were reported that their height were between 1.61-1.70 meters (40 respondents, figure 2), which is followed by the height intervals 1.81-1.90 meters (35 respondents, 26.95%), and 1.71-1.70 meters (34 respondents, 26.15%).

Table 1 shows the weight distribution of the respondents, where majority (33 respondents, 25.28%) of the respondents were 51-60 kilograms, and this was followed by 61-70 kilograms of the 25 respondents. It was observed that 4 of the 130 respondents were heavier than 100 kilograms, and 10 respondents were lighter than 50 kilograms.

The keyboard and mouse were reported to be the most popular (90.77%) input devices, whereas only 12 (9.23%) of the 130 respondents were using touchpad, keypad and trackball as primary input devices.

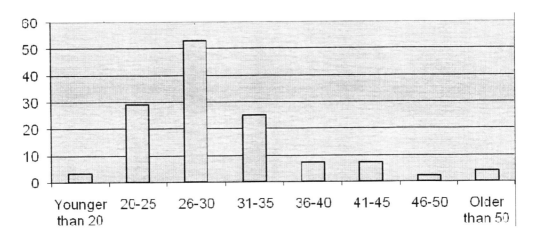

Figure 1. Distribution of age of the respondents.

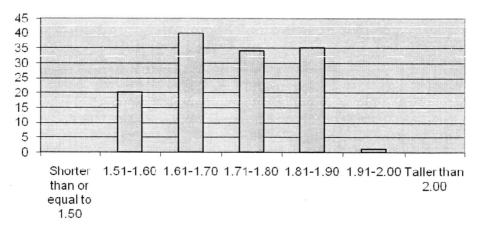

Figure2. Height distribution of the respondents.

Table 1. Weight distribution of the respondents

Weight	Number of Respondents	Percentage of Respondents
Less than or equal to 50	10	7.69%
51-60	33	25.38%
61-70	25	19.23%
71-80	23	17.69%
81-90	23	17.69%
91-100	12	9.23%
More than 100	4	3.08%

Moreover, 88.43% of the respondents were using regular (Q-type) keyboards, 3.31% were using F-type keyboards, and 4.96% were using ergonomic (with wrist support) keyboards. Additionally, 72.31% of the respondents were using desktop and 27.69% of the respondents were using laptop computers. Regarding the keyboard use, it was found that 55.04% of the respondents have been using keyboard for 10 or more years, and 37.98% have been using keyboard for at least 5 years (figure 3).

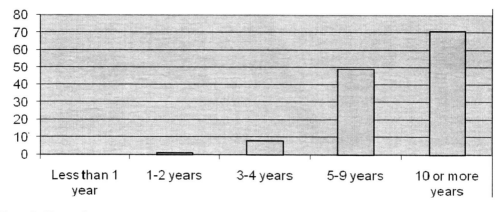

Figure 3. Years of computer use.

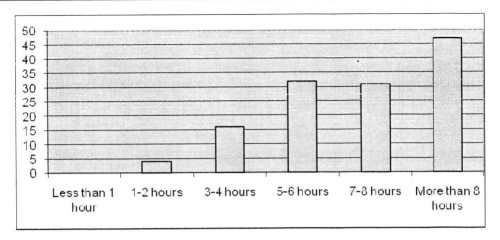

Figure 4. Daily keyboard uses.

Around 24.62% of the respondents reported their daily keyboard use as 5-6 hours per day, 23.85% of them as 7-8 hours per day, and 36.15% of them as more than 8 hours per day (figure 4).

The results of the questionnaire indicated that 79.84% of the respondents found their job interesting, where 20.16% of the respondents indicated that they did not find their job interesting. Additionally, 74.42% of the respondents mentioned that their job gives them personal satisfaction; however 25.58% of the respondents mentioned that they were not having personal satisfaction from their job.

A very high majority of the respondents (90.62%) reported that they have "good" relationship with their supervisor/advisor, where 9.38% reported that they have "not good" relationship with their supervisor/advisor.

More than two thirds of the respondents indicated that they share their office, where 35.66% share the office with more than three people, and 33.33% share the office with three or less people. On the other hand, 31.01% reported that they have their own office.

Majority of the respondents (84.38%) reported that they like their office environment, whereas 15.62% of the respondents reported that they do not like their office environment. Addition to this, a very high majority (94.57%) of the respondents indicated that they like working with computers, however only 5.43% of the respondents indicated that they do not like working with computers.

Most of the respondents (64.04%) reported that they have a stressful job, but 35.94% of the respondents reported that they do not have a stressful job. It was observed that, 48.84% of the respondents think that they have enough rest breaks, and 51.16% of the respondents do not think that they have enough rest breaks.

Additionally, 46.88% of the respondents have repetitive (static) jobs, whereas 53.12% of the respondents have non-repetitive (dynamic) jobs. Only 18.60% of the respondents were smoking when they answered the questionnaire, and 81.40% of the respondents were not smoking. More than half of the smoking respondents (63.41%) reported that they were smoking during the previous year, and 36.59% of the respondents were not smoking during the previous year. Table 2 shows the results obtained on the ergonomic qualities applied in the workstations.

Table 2. Office ergonomics qualities (*n* = 130)

Office Ergonomics	Yes (%)	No (%)
Lean back to support vertebrae	56.92	43.08
Elbows form 90 degrees from shoulder	41.54	58.46
Feet are comfortable in the front	67.69	32.31
Seat and hands are centered on the keyboard	81.54	18.46
Sit symmetrically	50.77	49.23
Keyboard and mouse are at the fingertips	79.23	20.77
Keyboard and mouse are at the same level	77.69	22.31
Screen is arm length away from the eyes	80.62	19.38
Monitor is at the eye level	65.38	34.62
Sufficient lightening available, no glare	72.87	27.13
Talk on phone between head and shoulder	26.36	73.64
Neutral wrist position	78.46	21.54
Neutral head and neck position	64.62	35.38
Elbow and arm support available	48.84	51.16
Leg support available	25.58	74.42
Change sitting position every 15 min	57.69	42.21
Take active breaks	55.38	44.62
Take frequent microbreaks	45.38	54.62
Trained in posture	21.54	78.46

The results show that 56.92% of the respondents lean back to support their vertebrae, 67.69% reported that their feet were comfortable in the front, 81.54% stated that their seat and hands were centered on the keyboard, more than half (50.77%) of the respondents sit symmetrically, 79.23% use keyboard and mouse at the fingertips, 77.69% have the keyboard and the mouse at the same level, 80.62% of the respondents' screens were about arm length away from their eyes, 65.38% had the monitors at the eye level, 72.87% had sufficient lightening without glare, 78.46% had neutral wrist position, and 64.62% had neutral head and neck position.

However, the majority of the respondents didn't take into consideration of having 90^0 angle between the shoulders and the elbows. They did not care about sitting symmetrically at all, and they usually (73.64%) talked on the phone by having the handset between the head and the shoulder. Elbow, arm or leg supports also were not available in the respondents' workstations. Moreover, the majority of the respondents (78.46%) were not trained in posture (table 2).

Table 3 shows that the most prevalent discomfort experienced was observed having ache in the neck (42.31%). Discomfort (feeling of pain) was observed to be the next prevalent discomfort after ache. It was reported by the respondents that 31.54% of them were experiencing pain in the neck. Tightness was reported by 10.77% of the respondents in the neck, and 10.00% of the respondents stated that they have a feeling of heaviness in the neck. Having cramp was reported by 7.69% of the respondents in the neck, and weakness in the neck was reported by 4.62%. Feeling of hot and cold was reported by 1.54% of the respondents and only 0.77% of them reported tingling and swelling in their necks. None of the respondents indicated that they experience symptoms of numbness in their necks.

Table 3. Type of discomfort and percent occurrence in the neck

	Percent Occurrence
Ache	42,31
Pain	31,54
Cramp	7,69
Tingling	0,77
Numbness	0,00
Heaviness	10,00
Weakness	4,62
Tightness	10,77
Feeling Hot and Cold	1,54
Swelling	0,77

Therefore, the discomfort feelings of ache and pain were the most common types of discomforts which are experienced at the neck.

It was reported by the respondents that they were having the discomforts in their neck sometimes 25.38%, often 23.08%, rarely 12.31%, and very often 10.77% (table 4).

Table 4. Frequency of discomfort

	Never (%)	Rarely (%)	Sometimes (%)	Often (%)	Very Often (%)
Neck	9.23	12.31	25.38	23.08	10.77

Among the 130 respondents, 17 had a recent accident and 6 of those had this accident within 12 months (4.62% of the whole population). Also, 23 respondents reported that they had diagnosed with a work-related musculoskeletal disorder by a medical doctor, and 11 (8.46% of the whole respondents) of the sufferers reported this diagnosis had been made within the last 12 months.

Additionally, 4 respondents (3.08%) reported that they were diagnosed with rheumatoid arthritis, 1 respondent (0.77%) with diabetes, 4 respondents (3.08%) with thyroid disease, 8 respondents (6.15%) with pinched nerve. Moreover, 3 respondents were pregnant and 14 respondents with other medical symptoms and none of the respondents reported that they were diagnosed with hemophilia.

It was reported by the respondents that, 41 (31.54%) of them exercise never/rarely, 57 (43.85%) sometimes, 25 (19.23%) often, and only 7 (5.38%) of them exercise very often. Moreover, 91 of the respondents (70%) stated that they were involved in sport activities, and 39 of them (30%) reported that they were not involved in any kind of sport activities.

More than half of the respondents (76, 58.46%) reported that they were involved in walking as sport activity, 17 of the respondents (13.08%) did jogging, 15 (11.54%) of them played football, 4 (3.08%) of them played basketball, 5 (3.85%) of them played volleyball, 10 (7.69%) of them played tennis, 26 (20.00%) did swimming, and 27 (20.77%) involved in other sport activities (figure 5).

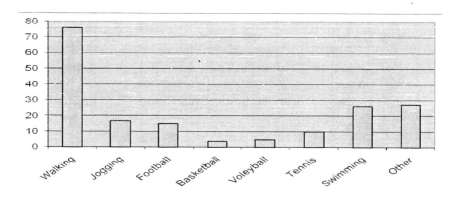

Figure 5. Sport activities involved.

3.2. Data Analysis

Logistic Regression Analysis is used to develop and to determine a meaningful and statistically significant relationship exists between work-related musculoskeletal disorders and computer use as a risk assessment model. The logistic regression was used because many of the independent variables were qualitative and the normality of residuals cannot be guaranteed. Table 5 shows that none of the above ergonomics factors are found to be significant predictors of WRMSDs in the neck for the collected data.

Table 5. Logistic Regression of Ergonomic Factors that affect the Neck

Predictor	Coef	SE Coef	Z	P	Odds Ratio	95% CI Lower	Upper
Constant	2.86623	1.23941	2.31	0.021			
Neutral head and neck position	-0.412071	0.536055	-0.77	0.442	0.66	0.23	1.89
Telephone use position	-0.642894	0.577044	-1.11	0.265	0.53	0.17	1.63

Table 6. Logistic Regression of Feelings of Discomforts in the Neck

Predictor	Coef	SE Coef	Z	P	Odds Ratio	95% CI Lower	Upper
Constant	3.67027	1.35714	2.70	0.007			
Ache	-0.767427	0.519816	-1.48	0.140	0.46	0.17	1.29
Pain	0.0495422	0.591109	0.08	0.933	1.05	0.33	3.35
Cramp	-0.101447	1.02564	-0.10	0.921	0.90	0.12	6.75
Tingling	21.6843	33701.2	0.00	0.999	2.61442E+09	0.00	*
Heaviness	-0.574743	0.818888	-0.70	0.483	0.56	0.11	2.80
Weakness	-0.0951334	1.50795	-0.06	0.950	0.91	0.05	17.47
Tightness	-0.0726508	0.839722	-0.09	0.931	0.93	0.18	4.82
Felling HotandCold	-1.54086	2.15630	-0.71	0.475	0.21	0.00	14.67
Swelling	21.2434	33701.2	0.00	0.999	1.68232E+09	0.00	*

Table 6 shows that none of the above feeling discomfort and ergonomics factors are found to be significant predictors of WRMSDs in the neck for the collected data.

Table 7 shows that rarely in the neck ($p=0.006<0.05$) and often in the neck ($p=0.010<0.05$) are found to be significant predictors of WRMSDs for the collected data.

Table 7. Logistic Regression of Frequency of Discomforts in the Neck

Predictor	Coef	SE Coef	Z	P	Odds Ratio	95% CI Lower	Upper
Constant	3.17873	0.832437	3.82	0.000			
Neck Never	-1.56929	1.13708	-1.38	0.168	0.21	0.02	1.93
Neck Rarely	-2.66790	0.979601	-2.72	0.006	0.07	0.01	0.47
Neck Sometimes	-1.07032	0.949120	-1.13	0.259	0.34	0.05	2.20
Neck Often	-2.24852	0.872157	-2.58	0.010	0.11	0.02	0.58
Neck Very Often	-1.10800	1.07452	-1.03	0.302	0.33	0.04	2.71

3.3. Experimental Results

After developing the risk assessment model, the model should be validated and be verified. Towards this end, we have to first identify those respondents under risk. Then, the data analysis of the surface EMG recordings is supposed to provide the validation and verification of the models fitted.

Odds ratios for each significant factor determined by the logistic regression analysis were calculated and those respondents who have higher odds ratios for each factor were identified.

It was observed that fifteen respondents were under risk of having WRMSDs according to the results of odds ratio analysis. However, only six of the fifteen respondents were able to be contacted and invited to the sEMG data collection experiment. That group of six respondents formed the test group, and among the non-risk respondent group, six more respondents were invited to form the control group.

In the sEMG experiment, muscular activity in the neck (posterior upper trapezius) was recorded by using sEMG device (MyoTrac Infiniti, model SA9800). The procedure for the experimentation is as follows; 20 minutes typing exercise was given to each respondent at a time. Data were collected at 5th, 10th, 15th, and 20th minutes of the experimentation. The mean value of the collected data for 30 seconds is then calculated and taken into consideration.

3.3.1. Test Group Experimental Results

The readings from sEMG provides the information about the muscle activity in the neck over time. Table 8 illustrates the mean value for each 30 seconds interval readings for each test group respondent.

The muscle activity is converted to µV by sEMG and is shown on the vertical line, and time is shown on the horizontal line in seconds (figure 6).

Figure 6 illustrates that test group respondents have significantly high levels of muscle activities. Test group respondent 1 has been suffering from discomforts at the neck very significantly more than in other 5 respondents. The test group respondents 5 and 6 have also muscle activities relatively more than the others.

Table 8. Muscle activities (µV) of the test group respondents at the neck

Muscle Activity	minutes			
Test Group	5	10	15	20
Respondent 1	2373.68	2770.17	2890.90	2729.68
Respondent 2	28.07	29.06	37.02	34.58
Respondent 3	92.56	79.05	61.78	50.86
Respondent 4	186.04	187.67	158.85	196.42
Respondent 5	911.45	758.30	972.51	455.92
Respondent 6	1158.83	567.27	584.80	471.55

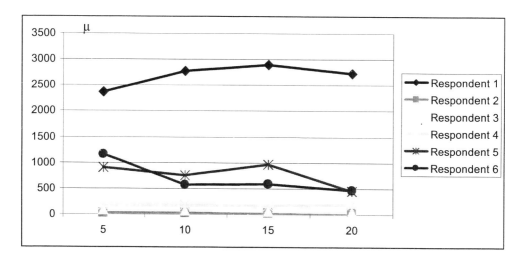

Figure 6. Muscle activity recordings in the neck of test group respondents.

$F_0 = 120.959 > F_{0.05,5,18} = 2.77$; therefore, reject H_o,

where;

H_0 = mean musculoskeletal strain (in time) of the 6 respondents does not differ, and
H_1 = mean musculoskeletal strain (in time) of the 6 respondents does not differs.

The results obtained by ANOVA indicate that, the risk assessment model developed has been validated and verified with the data collected through sEMG recordings.

3.3.2. Control Group Experimental Results

The control group respondents were selected among the group of respondents who were not under risk according to the odds ratios.

Table 9 illustrates the mean value for each 30 seconds interval sEMG readings for each control group respondent.

Figure 7 illustrates that control group respondents' muscle activities do not significantly differ from each other and these readings were not at high levels.

Table 9. ANOVA results for the test group respondents

Source of Variation	SS	df	MS	F	P-value	F crit
Between Groups	20278244	5	4055649	120.959	3.34E-13	2.772853
Within Groups	603524.2	18	33529.12			
Total	20881769	23				

Table 10. Muscle activities (µV) of the control group respondents at the neck

Muscle Activity	minutes			
Control Group	5	10	15	20
Respondent 1	20.91	67.62	59.55	27.82
Respondent 2	14.55	53.79	48.21	30.55
Respondent 3	28.22	77.33	26.73	19.27
Respondent 4	15.68	45.08	83.37	41.72
Respondent 5	22.55	69.30	137.65	119.40
Respondent 6	19.33	39.45	16.62	43.92

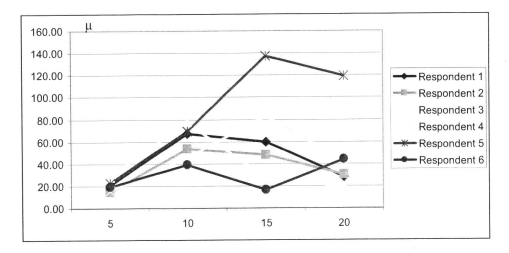

Figure 7: Muscle activity recordings in the neck of control group respondents

Table 11. ANOVA results for the control group respondents

Source of Variation	SS	df	MS	F	P-value	F crit
Between Groups	8440.443	5	1688.089	1.940491	0.13724	2.772853
Within Groups	15658.71	18	869.9286			
Total	24099.16	23				

$F_0 = 1.94 < F_{0.05, 5, 18} = 2.77$; therefore, fail to reject H_o,

where;

H_0 = mean musculoskeletal strain (in time) of the 6 respondents does not differ, and
H_1 = mean musculoskeletal strain (in time) of the 6 respondents does not differs.

The results of the ANOVA for each control group respondent indicate that, the mean musculoskeletal strain that they experience does not differ in time. That is, the musculoskeletal strain at their neck do not differ as those in the test group respondents.

ANOVA results for the control group respondents support the risk assessment model developed to determine the risk factors of WRMSDs.

CONCLUSION

Most of the studies on the formation of WRMSDs in human-computer interaction have been focused on the gender differences, physical and psychological aspects of the user and have not yet considered extra-rational factors such as the perceived musculoskeletal discomfort types and their frequencies. This study presents the idea of understanding how demographic structure, physical and psychosocial job characteristics, office ergonomics, perceived musculoskeletal discomfort types and their frequencies may affect formation of musculoskeletal disorders at the neck.

After collecting data from 130 respondents, the significant factors that would result in the development WRMSDs during computer use were predicted to be:

- Rarely in the neck [OR=0.07, CI: 0.01-0.0.47]
- Often in the neck [OR=0.11, CI: 0.02-0.58]

This study provided the evidence that, ache and pain are the most common types of the discomforts in the neck. Musculoskeletal strain has not the same effect on each the 6 respondents (from ANOVA) who were examined through sEMG.

REFERENCES

Amell, T. K., Kumar, S., 1999. Cumulative trauma disorders and keyboarding work. *International Journal of Industrial Ergonomics* 25, 69-78.

Aptel, M., Aublet-Cuvelier, A., Cnockaert, J. C., 2002. Work-related musculoskeletal disorders of the upper limb. *Joint Bone Spine* 69, 546-555.

Arocena, P., Núñez, I., Villanueva, M., 2008. The impact of prevention measures and organisational factors on occupational injuries. *Safety Science* 46 (9), 1369-1384.

Babski-Reeves, K. L., Crumtpon-Young, L. L, "Comparisons of measures for quantifying repetition in predicting carpal tunnel syndrome", *International Journal of Industrial Ergonomics*, 30(1): 1-6, 2002.

Balcı, R., Aghazadeh, F., 2003. The effect of work-rest schedules and type of task on the discomfort and performance of VDT users. *Ergonomics* 46 (3), 455-465.

Blatter, B. M., Bongers, P. M., 2002. Duration of computer use and mouse use in relation to musculoskeletal disorders of neck or upper limb. *International Journal of Industrial Ergonomics* 30, 295-306.

Buckle, P. W., Devereux J. J., 2002. The nature of work-related neck and upper limb musculoskeletal disorders. *Applied Ergonomics* 33, 207–217.

Carayon, P., Smith, M. J., Haims, M. C., "Work Organization, Job Stress, and Work-Related Musculoskeletal Disorders", *Human Factors*, 41 (4): 644-663, 1999.

Cook, C., Burgess-Limerick, R., Chang, S., 2000. The prevalence of neck and upper extremity musculoskeletal symptoms in computer mouse users. *International Journal of Industrial Ergonomics* 26 (3), 347-356.

Cooper, A., Straker, L., 1998. Mouse versus keyboard use: A comparison of shoulder muscle load. *International Journal of Industrial Ergonomics* 22, 351-357.

Editorial, 2002. Muscular disorders in computer users: introduction. *International Journal of Industrial Ergonomics* 30, 203-210.

Engkvist, Inga-Lill, 2008. Back injuries among nurses – A comparison of the accident processes after a 10-year follow-up. *Safety Science* 46 (2), 291-301.

Evans, O., Patterson, K., "Predictors of neck and shoulder pain in non-secretarial computer users", *International Journal of Industrial Ergonomics*, 26: 357-365, 2000.

Fagarasanu, M., Kumar, S., 2003. Carpal Tunnel Syndrome due to keyboarding and mouse tasks: a review. *International Journal of Industrial Ergonomics* 31 (2), 119-136.

Fogleman M., Lewis, R. J., 2002. Factors associated with self-reported musculoskeletal discomfort in video display terminal (VDT) users. *International Journal of Industrial Ergonomics* 29, 311-318.

Hair, J. F. Jr., Anderson, R. E., Tatham, R. L., Black, W. C. Multivariate Data Analysis: With Readings, Prentice Hall, February 1995, 4th edition.

Jensen, C., Finsen, L., Søgaard, K., Christensen, H., 2002. Musculoskeletal symptoms and duration of computer and mouse. *International Journal of Industrial Ergonomics* 30 (4-5), 265-275.

Karlqvist, L., Tornqvist, E. W., Magberg, M., Hagman, M., Toomingas, A., 2002. Self-reported working conditions of VDU operators and associations with musculoskeletal symptoms: a cross-sectional study focusing on gender differences. *International Journal of Industrial Ergonomics* 30, 277-294.

Korhan, Orhan. "*Association of Emotions and Musculoskeletal Stress in Computer Users: An Occupational Risk Assessment Modelling*". Lambert Academic Publishing, Germany 2010. ISBN: 978-3-8383-5525-2.

Korhan, Orhan. "*Work-Related Musculoskeletal Disorders due to Computer Use: A Literature Review*". Lambert Academic Publishing, Germany 2010. ISBN: 978-3-8383-6625-8.

Korhan, O., Mackieh A. 2010. A Model for Occupational Injury Risk Assessment of Musculoskeletal Discomfort and Their Frequencies in Computer Users. *Safety Science*, Vol. 48 (7), 868-877.

Korhan, O., Mackieh A. An empirical study on work related musculoskeletal disorders during computer use. *African Journal of Business Management* (February 2011).

Lewis, R. J., Krawiec, M., Confer, E., Agopsowicz, D., Crandall, E., 2002. Musculoskeletal disorder worker compensation costs and injuries before and after an office ergonomics program. *International Journal of Industrial Ergonomics* 29, 95-99.

Liao, M. H., Drury, C. G., 2000. Posture, discomfort and performance in a VDT task. *Ergonomics* 43 (3), 345-359.

Mekhora K., Liston, C. B., Nanthavanij, S., Cole, J. H., 2000. The effect of ergonomic intervention on discomfort in computer users with tension neck syndrome. International Journal of Industrial Ergonomics 26, 367,-379.

Matias, A. C., Salvendy, G., Kuczek, T., "Predictive models of carpal tunnel syndrome causation among VDT operators", *Ergonomics*, 41: 213-226, 1998.

Ming, Z., Zaproudina, N., 2003. Computer use related upper limb musculoskeletal (ComRULM) disorders. *Pathophysiology* 9, 155-160.

Palei, S. K., Das S. K., 2009. Logistic regression model for prediction of roof fall risks in bord and pillar workings in coal mines: An approach. *Safety Science* 47 (1), 88-96.

Peper, E., Wilson, V. S., Gibney, K. H., Huber, K., Harvey, R., Shumay, D., M., "The integration of electromyography (SEMG) at the workstation: assessment, treatment, and prevention of repetitive stain injury (RSI)", *Applied Psychophysiology and Biofeedback*, 28 (2): 167-182, 2003.

Press, S. J., Wilson, S., 1978. Choosing between Logistic Regression and Discriminant Ananlysis. *Journal of American Statistical Association* 73 (364), 699-705.

Punnett, L., Bergqvist, U., 1997. Visual Display Unit Work and Upper Extremity Musculoskeletal Disorders. *A Review of Epidemiological Findings*. National Institute for Working Life - Ergonomic Expert Committee Document No 1, 1997:16.

Shuval, K., Donchin, M., "Prevalence of upper extremity musculoskeletal symptoms and ergonomic risk factors at a High-Tech company in Israel", *International Journal of Industrial Ergonomics*, 35: 569-581, 2005.

Tittiranonda, P., Rempel, D., Armstrong, T., Burastero, S., 1999. Effect of four computer keyboards in computer users with upper extremity musculoskeletal disorders. *American Journal of Industrial Medicine* 35, 647-661.

Westgaard, R. H., 2000. Work-related musculoskeletal complaints: some ergonomics challenges upon the start of a new century. *Applied Ergonomics* 31, 569-580.

Van Duijne, R. H., Van Aken, D., Schouten, E. G., 2008. Considerations in developing complete and quantified methods for risk assessment. *Safety Science* 46 (2), 245-254.

In: Neck Pain: Causes, Diagnosis and Management
Editor: Gregorio Lombardi

ISBN 978-1-61470-363-1
© 2012 Nova Science Publishers, Inc.

Chapter 3

SUPPORT OF RSI: ROLFING STRUCTURAL INTEGRATION FOR REDUCING PAIN AND LIMITATIONS OF MOTION IN THE NECK AND SHOULDER

Helen James[1], Janice Brown[2], Annie Burke-Doe[3] and M. E. Miller[4]

[1]Adv Cert Rolfer; private practice, Clovis, CA, U. S.
[2]UMDNJ, Newark School of Public Health, NJ, U. S.
[3]University of St Augustine for Health Sciences, San Diego, U. S.
[4]University of St Augustine for Health Sciences, San Diego, U. S.

ABSTRACT

Background. Misalignments in the body compromise the architectural integrity. At the tissue level, fascia shortens and thickens as the body engages in compensatory strategies to maintain itself upright, these changes are known as myofascial contractions. Fascia is found all over the body; therefore, when the fascia is altered, the movement capacity is decreased. Dupuytren disease, plantar fibromatosis, club foot, and frozen shoulder are examples of fascial disorders. In physical therapy, there are several methods by which practitioners treat these dysfunctions. However, studies showing the effect of those techniques are limited. *Purpose.* The purpose of studies by Brown (2010) and James, et al (2007) was to investigate the effect of Rolfing Structural Integration (RSI) in either shoulder or neck motion and pain levels of subjects who received RSI from a clinician who was both licensed in physical therapy and had advanced certification in RSI. RSI is a type of therapy that focuses on aligning the human body with gravity. Methods. This retrospective study reported by James et al over a period of years of clinical practice, analyzes changes in motion and pain levels at the neck for subjects who completed the RSI 10 basic sessions. Participants were evaluated before and after they received RSI. The data collected included: age, sex, occupation, referral source, diagnosis, height, weight, photographs of postural views, range of motion (ROM), pain, and functional complaints. ROM was assessed with the use of an arthordial protractor. Data analysis using three-way ANOVA tested the hypothesis at significance of 0.5.

Brown J, (2010) replicated the study using the same clinical data set for the shoulder. Results. The mean *pain* levels and *AROM* before RSI, significantly changed after the treatment (p < 0.5), there was a decrease in *pain* and an increase in *AROM*. *Pain Levels/AROM-Age* within subject effect demonstrated significant difference in *pain at best;* the mean pain levels in the older group decreased by 67%, and the mean AROM for in the younger group increased by 34 %. *Discussion.* In this sample: *Pain now* was reduced more than *pain best* and *pain worst*. Increased motion was reported for groups in both the neck and shoulder studies. *Conclusion*. This investigation demonstrates that the basic 10 sessions of RSI, when applied by a physical therapist with advanced RSI certification, decreases pain and increases AROM in adult subjects male and female with complaints of cervical spine or shoulder dysfunction regardless of age.

Keywords: RSI, Rolfing, motion, pain, neck, shoulder, physical therapy.

For the first time in more than a decade, the American Society of Anesthesiologists Task Force on Chronic Pain Management has updated its chronic pain guidelines. "The major change with this guideline is the fact that the guideline is developed from the perspective of interventions used to treat chronic pain," lead study author Richard Rosenquist, MD, from the University of Iowa Hospital, Iowa City, said in an interview. "Instead of looking at how to treat a given diagnosis, such as low back pain, the guideline examines the evidence to support the use of a broad range of interventions to treat chronic pain."The new guidelines appear in the April 2010 issue of *Anesthesiology*. The objectives are to optimize pain control, enhance physical and psychological well-being, and minimize adverse outcomes [Medscape CME 2011].

The role of the fascia in therapeutic interventions has been considered by practitioners of acupuncture, massage, structural integration [SI/RSI], chiropractic and osteopathy. But evidence based practice is limited, while many practitioners of these techniques work with the fascia data gathering, use of quantitative methods, and the research designs have been ignored; the reason researchers are now investigating this tissue. Fascia studies have considerably increased in the past few years, a Medline search 2004-7 indicated that in the last 3-4 years, titles or abstracts with the word "fascia" increased by more than 600% from the prior 4 to 18 years. Although the fascia is being studied in laboratories and clinics, there is still a strong need for further clinical exploration of this tissue [2].

Beginning in 2007 International Fascia Research Congresses have been held, with the third congress planned for March 2012. These gatherings of researchers span the range of research venues from current and retrospective reviews of clinical practice to controlled laboratory studies. The growth of literature in this previously ignored tissue is enlightening the interdisciplinary communities of physical medicine, physical therapy, body work and pain management as never before. Clinical interventions that seek to target this tissue to relieve pain and improve movement and posture are often labeled structural integration, and body work; as well as specific adaptations of the original intervention protocols that may be recognized by specific other names. These varied, and philosophically different techniques, are believed to have a common origin in the early 20th century Rolf Structural Integration (RSI) theories and practice by Ida P. Rolf, PhD.

In the 1920's Dr. Ida P. Rolf, after graduating from Columbia University with a Ph.D. in biochemistry, developed a holistic method of interventions that incorporate soft tissue manipulation and movement training for the purpose to facilitate the activities of daily living.[3]

Dr. Rolf's interest in the characteristics and function of collagen was the subject of her dissertation, as well as in her work as a research fellow at the Rockefeller Institute. Her work evolved into the Rolf Structural Integration (RSI) methods. RSI is a type of soft tissue mobilization therapy that focuses on aligning and balancing the body with gravity to maximize functional levels.[1-J] Rolf technique repositions the components of the human body in a vertical alignment so that the head, shoulder, thorax, pelvis and legs are aligned with gravity. [3,4,5] Thus when the body is structurally integrated, the force of gravity is controlled properly; therefore, the body's need of energy is decreased, and the movement capacity is improved [4,5] and pain decreases to allow for improved functional activities.

Dr. Rolf believed that when the internal structures are out of place, the body fights against gravity:

"some individuals may perceive their losing fight with gravity as a sharp pain in their back, others as the unflattering contour of their body, others as a constant fatigue; yet others as an unrelentingly threatening environment. Those over 40 may call it "old age." And yet these signals may be pointing to a single problem, so prominent in their own structure, as well as others, that is has been ignored: they are off balance. They are all at war with gravity." Ida P. Rolf Ph. D.[3]

Brown, J. 2010 states: "Rolfing Structural Integration (RSI) is a type of bodywork developed by Dr. Ida Rolf, Ph.D. biochemist, using concepts from osteopathic medicine and other manual therapies to develop an organized approach to analyzing and adjusting tension in the body's fascial layers. The basic premise of structural integration is that the body is organized in space and in the gravitational field, especially the upright position. The components of the body must be in proper distribution and balance for economical movement with minimal stress. As a result of physical trauma or emotional stress muscles and other tissues become displaced with compensatory adaptations of other muscles and fascial connections, often at distant points in the body. Through shortening and thickening of connective tissue and habitual patterns of movement, these muscular changes become chronic and involuntary."

James, et al (2007) state factors such as poor posture, injury, or stress, can contribute to misalignments in the body, which in turn, compromise its architectural integrity. At the tissue level, fascia shortens and thickens as the body engages in compensatory strategies to maintain itself upright, these changes are known as myofacial contractions [3].

Fascia is a type of tissue that creates continuity throughout the body. It is found in and around all the cells in the body, including myofibrils and all the organs. It is believed that fascia is the 'organ of form', because it is essential in the postures and the patterns of human movements. [6] The fascia contains the anatomical structures that give shape, form, stability and support to the body; so that when forces are applied to one point, they can be distributed to be absorbed by the entire body [3] Fascia makes up the aponeuroses, the joint capsules, and wraps the muscles as the endo-, peri and epimysium, [6,7] and extends as tendons, sharpey fibers, and periosteoum. It also forms the retinacula when it thickens transversally across bones to prevent tendons from expanding out of place during muscle activity; an example is found at the carpal tunnel [7].

The fascinating structure and movement of this tissue can be found in "Strolling Under the Skin" which was produced by a French plastic surgeon. This breathtaking in vivo video of fascia actions is available via www.anatomytrains.com

The superficial fascia is located under the skin, and facilitates skin movement and temperature regulation. The deep fascia is denser and highly organized [7] It creates compartments for groups of muscles that perform specific movements, and prevents the spreading and expanding out of the muscle during contraction [7,8] When the deep fascia deteriorates, it may lose its ability to limit expansion, allowing structural changes, such as varicose veins [8]. Therefore, when the structure of the fascia is altered, stiffness or weakness of the muscles can be experienced. Moreover, when the internal structures are altered, their intra- and intermuscular facial sheets lose their ability to slide over one another, and therefore, movement is decreased [2] Dupuytren disease, plantar fibromatosis, club foot, and frozen shoulder are examples of changes in the structure of the connective tissue/collagen [6].

Trauma to the fascia makes it thicker and shorter by positioning new connective tissue in a random manner. Inflammation due to repetitive use causes the connective tissue to be aligned with the lines of force in a fashion that compromises the biomechanics of the system [3,9,10]. These changes produce pain and stiffness. *"Some may describe these feelings as being tied up in knots; others as low energy; and of course, these feelings may be reflected in the mental state of the individual"- Ida P. Rolf.* RSI focuses on teaching the body to move in a more efficient and effective way by reversing strain and rigidity, while increasing its potential [3].

In Rolfing, practitioners employ a sequence of soft tissue manipulation techniques designed to enhance the symmetry and the balance of the human structure. They work on the fascia and connective tissue with their fingers, open hands, clenched fists and elbows [4] The pressure they apply is directed to release the adhesions between what should be sliding structures [2]. The quantity of pressure they apply, determines the amount of myofacial release and depends on the patient's ability to allow the change [11] Practitioners of this technique believe that contractures in the fascia do not have to be permanent changes because the chemical alterations of the matrix that are made of connective tissue can be rearranged so that collagen fibers can move again [2] Rolf practitioners apply the collagen alignment concepts to fascia structure and function [6]. They believe that improvements to the structure of the human body directly correlate with improvements in physiological and psychological functioning, [3,12] and that fascia adapts to physical stress, so that when they press against tissue, fascia changes its density, tonus or organization [6].

The 10 sessions of RSI modify asymmetries of standing postures by mobilizing the myofascial tissues [2] Sessions are individualized based upon the integrity of the soft tissue palpated, the posture observed and measured, and individual's complaints of dysfunction.[13] Research studies on RSI are few however the ones that have been conducted demonstrated considerable benefits on various physiological levels. The effect of pressure on collagen is documented by various authors:

Moyer's meta-analysis of massage therapy research [14] which included structural integration, showed single sessions of massage therapy achieving effect sizes of .3 to .4 SD on state anxiety, blood pressure and heart rate. Multiple sessions of massage showed higher effect sizes of .75 on anxiety and .62 on depression, providing benefits similar in magnitude to those of psychotherapy.

Deutsch, et al, [15] reported the use of RSI for the treatment of chronic pain. 20 subjects with chronic pain in the low back, cervical region, extremities, and other area demonstrated significant (p=0.05) improvements in ROM, posture, pain, and function. They reported a 74% decrease in pain and an increase of 85% in ROM.

Cottingham [12], et al documented the effects of RSI on the pelvic inclination angle and parasympathetic tone on 32 subjects with anterior tilted pelvis. They measured the inclination of the pelvis with an inclinometer, and the autonomic tone was reduced from the heart rate. Their results indicated significant decreases in standing anterior pelvic tilt immediately after the treatment and 24 hours after the treatment, and increased vagal tone in the subjects immediately after they received myofacial manipulation of the iliopsoas, deep hip rotators, and the hamstrings (p<0.01). There are two possible clinical applications to their findings. RSI can be used to treat low back pain associated with anterior tilt of the sacral base and the pelvis, and musculoskeletal disorders associated with autonomic stress disorders. Increases in vagal tone correlate with decreases in sympathetic nervous system activity, suggesting the use of RSI for treatment of autonomic dysfunctions. A randomized controlled study of structural integration showed that a single 45-minute session in 16 men who had previously had the ten-session treatment, resulted in increased heart rate variability, which persisted for 24 hours. The effect size was 1 SD immediately after the session, dropping to .75 SD 24 hours later. [12]

Weinberg, et.al., was concerned about the opinion of RSI practitioners and their clients regarding release of emotional tension stored up in the muscle in patients after RSI. His research team analyzed the means for state anxiety questionnaire scores before RSI and five weeks after RSI. There were 24 subjects assigned to the control group and 24 subjects in the experimental group. A significant decrease in anxiety in subjects who received RSI was reported (p<0.01). [4]

Perry, et.al., looked at functional effects of Rolfing on cerebral palsy. Ten patients diagnosed with cerebral palsy, aged from 10 to 42 years old received the 10 sessions of RSI. The analysis of the data revealed that subjects with mild impairments improve gait velocity, stride length and cadence, while subjects with moderate impairments slightly improved gait velocity. The researchers also noted increased tightness in the muscle of the hip and plantar flexors [2].

The 2007 RSI study by James et al supports the expected clinical correlation between pain and ROM: the more pain that subjects feel, the less likely that they will move [27] When the body posture is out of alignment, the fascia alters to compensate for changes in the redistribution of forces within the body [3] These changes in force distribution decrease the gliding properties of structures such as muscles, tendons, and nerves [2] that ultimately may promote entrapment or squeezing of pain receptors as the joints are moved. Therefore, application of RSI may decrease pain in the neck by preventing nerves from being squeezed or overstretched as a result of decreasing tension in the surrounding fascia. Increases in AROM may be attributed to a decrease in tension of the fascia and contractile tissue, allowing restoration of resting muscle length, thus restoring normal AROM and decreasing pain.

When muscles are in a sustained contraction, blood flow is restricted, cells become poorly supplied with cell nutrients, waste products are not eliminated properly, and free nerve endings are excited. These changes ultimately may manifest as pain [16] Tissue becomes nourished during activity and through tissue mobilization by the mechanical action that squeezes blood in and out of the vessels in the tissue. Mechanical skillful treatment of the soft tissue of the neck promotes circulation by relaxing the muscles, hence increasing blood flow and decreasing pain.

Older people are set apart from younger people by reductions in enzymes and fibers that regulate the biology, anatomy, and physiology of the body. In young people the fascia is properly hydrated maintaining its strength and flexibility; while in older people, it becomes thicker and firm as the collagen and elastin fibers increase their density, [17] hence, making it more difficult to release the fascia in older people. However when a physical therapist certified in RSI applied the Basic 10 Series, in studies of neck pain [27] (James,et al) and shoulder pain [19] (Brown) no significant findings by age or gender were reported. Finding in both studies were significant for decreased pain and increased movement, as well as improved or restored postural alignment of the body as a whole.

> Hunt, V. H., further illustrates myofascial contractions [18]
> Today there are numerous manipulative programs like rolfing, and exercises, which loosen and relax the connective tissues of the body. Now we know that connective tissue has piezoelectric capacities, which can act like an electrical system, where stretching enhances the electrical capacity. Therefore, we conjectured that connective tissue was more than tissue scaffolding. It seemed to dictate the flow of electromagnetic energy throughout the body at the fitness level.
> Dr. Valerie Hunt in a second randomized controlled trial found that Spielberger State Anxiety in 24 subjects improved from 39.4 ± 10 to 32.0 ± 8 after 10 sessions of Structural Integration, compared to 24 controls who went from 32.5 to 34.5 in the same time period.[5] This effect size of 0.7 SD was significant p<0.01 and is comparable to the effect sizes reported by Moyer.[14]

Brown (2010) [19] states that further support for the benefits of RSI can be explained by muscle physiology: when muscles are contracted, blood flow is restricted thus depriving muscle cells of nutrients and preventing proper elimination of waste products. The cellular waste products can in turn irritate nerve endings which manifests as pain. Thus, by releasing contracted muscles via their surrounding fascia, blood flow can resume, waste products removed, and nerve endings will be less irritated.

In addition to confirming a role for RSI in the management of people with shoulder dysfunction, the 2010 study by Brown [19] supports the expected clinical correlation between shoulder pain and shoulder AROM: the more pain that subjects feel the less likely they are to move their shoulder. What James et al explained in terms of the pathophysiology of cervical spine dysfunction and the hypothesized effect of RSI in that study can be applied to shoulder dysfunction: "When the [shoulder] is out of alignment with the body posture, the fascia alters to compensate for changes in the redistribution forces within the body [3]. These changes decrease the gliding properties of structures such as muscles, tendons, and nerves [2] that ultimately may promote entrapment or compression of pain receptors as the joints are moved. Thus, RSI may decrease pain in the [shoulder] by preventing nerves from being compressed or overstretched as a result of decreasing tension in the surrounding fascia. Increases in AROM may be attributed to a decrease in tension of the fascia and contractile tissue allowing restoration of resting muscle length. These findings suggest that RSI offers another solution in the treatment of movement dysfunction and warrants further investigation.

Helga Pohl, PhD in "*Changes in the structure of collagen distribution in the skin by a manual technique*" (2010) states: "in a practice of body therapy one encounters many persons with chronic complaints referred as sensory motor disorders. These individuals report sensations of pain, visceral symptoms, and movement disorders. The basis of these disorders are bodily impairments that can be palpated as changes in qualities of muscles, trigger points or connective tissue adjacent to the skin. These individuals can pinpoint the site/s of their discomfort. Qualitative changes in the underlying structures can be palpated at these sites." [20]

In addition to the site of complaint, additional areas may have qualitative changes as well. These identified areas have 'oversensitivity to pressure' compared to unaffected areas of the person. Dr Pohl studied this palpable difference using diagnostic ultrasound measures before and after soft tissue manipulation of the areas of qualitative difference. The findings supported the palpable differences; a reduction in density of the collagen distribution. Pohl speculates about the causes of this change in tissue quality; she supposes relaxation of the fibroblasts and increase in microcirculation. In the work by multiple researchers fibroblasts have been shown to form a network that exerts active mechanical foreces in many fascial tissues like subcutis, muscle fascia, and dermis. "Fibroblasts of the skin are able to contract collagen lattices and that their ability to contract can be changed by various substances." Pohl states "Relaxation of the fibroblasts and increased microcirculation may lead to (immediate) clinical phenomena of:

Less restricted movement
Reddening and swelling
Sensations of softness and warmth
Feelings of wellbeing
Pohl calls for further research on the duration of the immediate effects, and potential contributions to healing processes." [20]

Defining Pain [21]

Burke-Doe (2007) provides evidence of the multidimensional aspects of pain and multi-modal interventions to be considered. Pain is a sensation with more than one dimension. The primary purpose of pain is protective to the body. Pain occurs whenever there is tissue damage and it signals the individual to react to attempt to remove the painful stimulus. To the individual pain is both a subjective and objective experience. The objective dimension is the physiological tissue damage causing the pain. The subjective dimensions of pain include[22] the following:

- An affective component: the psychological factors surrounding the person's pain experience; including personality and emotional state.
- A behavioral component: how the person expresses the pain to others through communication and behavior.
- A cognitive component: what the person knows and believes about pain resulting from cultural background and past pain experiences of self and those of others in pain.

- A perceptual component: the personal awareness of the location, quality, intensity, and duration of the pain stimulus.

All of these dimensions of the sensations taken together constitute the personal pain experience; thus all dimensions must be addressed for a successful pain management program. When the subjective components are ignored, it may be possible to resolve the tissue damage without changing the person's perception pain.

Recognizing that pain is more than a physical injury or pathology helps health professionals explain some of the inconsistencies observed in patients with chronic pain. To select the most appropriate interventions clinicians need a general idea of pain pathways anatomy and physiology. The fact that pain transmission involves several higher centers of the nervous system that are interconnected help lead to resolution for some of the following common questions: [21] Why is one person's pain report out of proportion to the magnitude and duration of the injury? Why is pain intolerable to one person and merely uncomfortable to another? Why for the same individual, is the same or similar pain report tolerable at one time, yet is overwhelming at another time?

Categorizing Pain [21]

Pain descriptions may be grouped into several categories: acute, chronic, referred, autonomic, peripheral and neuropathic.

- *Acute pain* serves as a warning, it is localized, a physiological response that alerts the individual that the tissues are exposed to damaging stimuli.
- *Chronic pain* is defined as pain that continues after the stimulus is removed or tissue damage has healed. The pain for six months or more, is poorly localized, has an ill-defined onset, and is strongly associated with the subjective components of pain dimensions stated previously.
- *Referred pain* is felt at other than the point of origin. This pain could be stimulated by an internal organ, a joint, a trigger point, or a peripheral nerve; but is perceived as pain in a remote anatomical structure or location. This pain results from the convergence of primary afferent neurons from the structure of origin with the secondary neurons that also have a cutaneous receptive field. autonomic, peripheral and neuropathic.
- *Autonomic pain* may occur when the balance between afferent input and descending sympathetic systems are disrupted with injury, resulting in exaggerated and prolonged pain response; complex regional pain syndrome (CRPS) serves as an example of this category.
- *Peripheral pain* results from irritation of nociceptors, character of this pain is dependent upon location and intensity of stimulation, as well as the pain pathway stimulated.
- *Neuropathic pain* results from abnormal activity within the CNS [23], the involvement of the nervous system can be at many levels. This pain is distinct from nociceptive pain (non-neuronal tissue damage).

Persistent pain is now considered to have a psychogenic component [24]. The multidimensional aspects of pain indicate the significance of evaluation of the causative nature as well as the emotional and cognitive sequel [25]. Many emotional factors can strongly influence pain. The emotional experience that we perceive with pain reflects the interaction of higher neurological centers. The physical limitations of pain are commonly assessed, it is the *mind-body connection* that is less often articulated by the person in pain, and an area more difficult for the clinician. Patient-centered models such as the International Classification of Functioning, Disability and Health (ICF) provides a framework to acknowledge the multidimensional nature of complaints of pain, yet lead to interventions that improve physical functional activities, while providing cognitive and behavioral strategies to help in resuming activities of daily life.

Examination of persons with complaints of pain requires *a comprehensive pain history*. [21] Such a pain history would include: *Observation* from entry to the service site, through examination, and continues until the person exits the service site. Pain *origin/onset circumstances* should be documented. *Position:* location of the pain by demonstration from the individual seeking services. *Pattern* of the complaint; document the reported characteristics of the pain. *Quality*: what terms are used to describe the sensation? i.e. burning, traveling, stabbing, etc. *Quantity*: intensity of the sensation. There are valid and reliable measures for quantifying this information in documentation for both adults and children. *Radiation*: presence, absence, cause, of this sensation. *Signs/symptoms*: how does the sensation interfere with the person's lifestyle? *Treatment*: what interventions has the person experienced prior to this examination? *Visceral symptoms*: which of these complaints accompany the pain.

Burke-Doe highlights three broad areas to include in *pain management intervention*. [21] Each area addresses a different aspect of the pain experience and each area requires a different level of participation from the person with pain. The three areas of intervention are: physical activity and modalities, cognitive strategies, and behavioral manipulations. These three interventions address the functional losses associated with the impairments, including the pain. The focus is on improving the function of the individual; preventing or resolving disability from the causative impairment as well as the resulting or accompanying pain response. Rolf Structural Integration Basic 10 Series as applied by a physical therapist with Advanced RSI Certification, demonstrates statistically significant findings for resolution of each complaint of cervical or shoulder pain and motion limitations of these two related anatomical regions as is reported in two independent studies of the shoulder [19] (Brown,2010) and of the neck [27] by James, et al(2007). Further research on the effects of RSI interventions for functional complaints in other areas of the body, rendered by practitioners with varied backgrounds, and to substantiate observational analysis are encouraged.

REFERENCES

[1]   Medscape CME Chronic Pain 2010
[2]   Findley TW, and Shleip R. *Fascia research. Basic science and implication for conventional and complementary health care.* Germany. Elsevier; 2007:2-3.

[3] Findley T, DeFilippis J. Information for clinical health care practitioners. *Rolfing Structural Integration - The Rolf Institute Research Committee.* 2005;October 1-6.

[4] Perry J, Jones MH, Thomas, L. Functional evaluation of Rolfing in cerebral palsy. *Develop. Med. Child Neurol.* 1981;23:717-729.

[5] Weinberg, RS, Hunt VV. Effects of structural integration on state-strait anxiety. *Journal of Clinical Psychology.* 1979;35:319-322.

[6] Schleip R. Fascial plasticity – a new neurobiological explanation: part 1. *Journal of body bodywork and movement therapies.* 2003; 7:11-19.

[7] Levangie PK, Nokin CC. *Joint structure and function.* United States: Davis Company; 2000:93-94.

[8] Moore, KL, Dalley AF. *Clinical oriented anatomy.* New York: Lippincott Williams and Wilkins; 1999:522, 526, 998.

[9] Godman CC, Boissonnault WG, Fuller KS. *Pathology, implication for the physical therapist.* New York: Saunders; 2003:1147-1150.

[10] O'sullivan SB, Schmitz, TJ. *Physical rehabilitation, assessment and treatment.* Philadelphia, PA: F. A. Davis; 2001:682.

[11] Fahey, B. *The power of balance: A Rolfing view of health.* Portland, Oregon: Metamorphous Press; 1989:8-175-176.

[12] Cottingham JT, Porges SW, Richmond, K. Shift inclination angle and parasympathetic tone produced by rolfing soft tissue manipulation. *Journal of American Physical Therapy Association.* 1988; 68:1364-1370.

[13] Kuchars D J, Swan C. Discover the rhythms. *American fitness.* 1992;10: 40-43.

[14] Moyer CA, Rounds J, Hannum JW A Metal Analysis of Massage Therapy Research Psychol Bull.130: 3-18, 2004.

[15] Deutsch JE, Derr LL, Judd P, Reuven B. Treatment of chronic pain through the use of structural integration (Rolfing). *Orthopaedic Physical Therapy Clinics of North America.* 2000. 9(3): 411-27.

[16] Cailliet R. *Neck and arm pain.* F. A. Davis Company. Philadelphia:1981;42-43.

[17] Bottomley CL. *Geriatric rehabilitation: A clinical approach.* Upper Saddle River, NJ: Prentice-Hall: 2003:50-54, 61.

[18] Hunt, VH. *The science of human vibration.* Malibu, CA: Malibu Publishing Company; 1995:12.

[19] Brown, J., unpublished paper 2010: Retrospective Outcome Study of Rolfing Structural Integration for Shoulder Pain and Active Range of Motion.

[20] Pohl, H. "Changes in the structure of collagen distribution in the skin caused by a manual technique" Available from:www.sciencedirect.com/jbmt (2010)14,27-34 Elsevier.

[21] Burke-Doe A; Pain Management. In: Umphred, D., et al editors. *Neurological Rehabilitation* 5th ed; St. Louis, Mo.: Mosby, Inc an affiliate of Elsevier, 2007; 1036-1060.

[22] Nolan MF; Pain: the experience and its expression. *Clin Management* 10:22, 1990.

[23] Borsook D, LeBel A, Stojanovic M et al; Central pain syndromes. In Ashburn, MA, editor: The management of pain. New York, 1988. Churchill Livingston.

[24] Weatherley CR, Prickett CF, O'Brien JP; Discogenic pain persisting despite solid posterior fusion. *J Bone Joint Surg Br* 68: 142-143, 1986.

[25] Summers JD, Rapoff MA, Varghese G et al; Psychosocial factors in chronic spinal cord injury pain, *Pain* 47: 183-189, 1991.
[26] Steiner WA, Ryser L, Huber E et al; Use of the ICF model as a clinical problem-solving tool in physical therapy and rehabilitation medicine. *Phys Ther* 82:1098-1107, 2002.
[27] James H, Castaneda L, Miller ME, Findley T. Rolfing structural integration treatment of cervical spine dysfunction. *J Bodywork and Movement Therapies* (September 2008).

In: Neck Pain: Causes, Diagnosis and Management
Editor: Gregorio Lombardi

ISBN 978-1-61470-363-1
© 2012 Nova Science Publishers, Inc.

Chapter 4

NECK PAIN INDUCED BY DEEP NECK INFECTIONS

Masahiro Nakayama, Keiji Tabuchi and Akira Hara*
Department of Otolaryngology
Graduate School of Comprehensive Human Sciences
University of Tsukuba
Tsukuba, Japan

ABSTRACT

Neck pain is often caused by numerous spinal problems including inflammation, muscular tightness in both the neck and upper back, and pinching of the nerves emanating from the cervical vertebrae. Various head and neck lesions such as neck infections also induce neck pain. Most deep neck infections were caused by spreading from pharyngeal and odontogenic origins, and induce marked neck pain. Since they may rapidly compromise the airway, and also spread to the mediastinum or cause sepsis, a lack of awareness of these conditions and a delayed diagnosis may lead to potentially fatal consequences. This review discusses the causes, evaluation, and available treatments for the common type of neck pain induced by infections in head and neck regions. Early diagnosis and treatment are essential in order to prevent life-threatening complications.

INTRODUCTION

Neck pain, being a common complaint, can be caused by injury, stress, or by other health problems, including some that may cause serious consequences. The following medical conditions are some of the possible causes considered in the patients with neck pain:

---

* Address for correspondence: Keiji Tabuchi, Department of Otolaryngology. Graduate School of Comprehensive Human Sciences. University of Tsukuba. 1-1-1 Tennodai, Tsukuba 305-8575, Japan. TEL: +81-298-53-3147. FAX: +81-298-53-3147. E-mail: ktabuchi@md.tsukuba.ac.jp

- Neck injury
- Whiplash
- Neck strain
- Neck muscle disorder
- Neck muscle spasm
- Neck ligament disorder
- Torticollis
- Spinal disorder
- Arthritis
- Rheumatoid arthritis
- Cervical spondylosis
- Disc disorders
- Carotidynia
- Congenital cervical rib
- Cervical spine infection
- Swollen neck lymph nodes
- Head and neck infection
- Head and neck cancers

Deep neck infection is an infection in the potential spaces and fascial planes of the neck, either with abscess formation or cellulitis, and induces severe neck pain in many cases. The incidence of this disease was relatively high before the advent of antibiotics. Antibiotics resulted in a significant decrease in the occurrence and the progression of this disease. However, when not diagnosed and treated appropriately, these infections progress rapidly and are still associated with high morbidity and mortality (Suehara et al., 2008). The potential serious complications of deep neck infection include airway obstruction, jugular vein thrombosis, aneurysm or rupture of the carotid artery, mediastinitis, and sepsis. Although antibiotic therapy has improved the outcome of deep neck infections, surgery is often necessary for drainage, especially as these infections, caused by bacteria that are resistant to many antibiotics, become increasingly common (Barlett et al., 1995; Coonan et al., 1994).

In order to successfully diagnose and treat patients with neck pain caused by deep neck infections, an understanding of deep neck infections, their common etiologies, typical presentation, clinical course, and so on is mandatory. In this chapter, diagnosis and management of deep neck infections are discussed.

NECK SPACES

Before considering deep neck infections, neck spaces are described. An understanding of the layers of the cervical fascia can help in determining the anatomic location of a deep neck infections, in predicting the extent of the infection, and in choosing an approach for surgical drainage. The cervical fascia is fibrous connective tissue that envelopes muscles and neurovascular bundles, dividing the neck and creating potential spaces. The two major divisions of the cervical fascia are the superficial and the deep (Cummings, 2005). The superficial fascia is located immediately below the dermis. It ensheathes the platysma and the muscles of facial expression. The deep cervical fascia is further divided into three layers: superficial, middle, and deep. All three layers of the deep cervical fascia contribute to consisting of the carotid sheath, enabling some deep neck infections to track to the great vessels of the neck and, from there, into the skull or the chest (Cummings, 2005; Crespo et al., 2004). The layers of the cervical fascia create potential spaces that can be occupied by infection. These spaces can be categorized by location as being: (1) in the face: the masticator, buccal, and parotid spaces; (2) in the suprahyoid neck: the peritonsillar, submandibular, sublingual, and parapharyngeal spaces; (3) in the infrahyoid neck: the anterior visceral space and; (4) extending the length of the neck: the retropharyngeal, danger space, prevertebral, and carotid sheath spaces (Chow, 1992).

(1) Face

The masticator space contains all four of the muscles of mastication: the medial and lateral pterygoid, masseter, and temporalis muscles. It also includes the ramus of the mandible and the third division of the trigeminal nerve. This space extends superiorly to the skull base and temporal fossa. The most common lesion in this space is an odontogenic abscess.

The buccal space has no true fascia boundaries and can be involved with processes extending from the masticator space such as tumor or infection. The buccinator muscles and the superficial muscles of facial expression border the buccal space. It contains mostly fat as well as minor salivary glands, the facial artery and veins, and the parotid duct.

The parotid space consists mainly of the parotid gland as well as portions of the facial nerve, retromandibular vein, and external carotid artery. There are also intraparotid and periparotid lymph nodes.

(2) Suprahyoid Neck

The submandibular space is located inferior to the mandible, between the mylohyoid muscles and the hyoid bone. This space contains the submandibular gland, submandibular and submental lymph nodes, the digastric muscles, facial veins , and fat.

The sublingual space is located within the oral cavity superior to the mylohyoid muscles. It contains the hyoglossus muscle, hypoglossal and lingual nerves, lingual artery and veins, sublingual gland, and a portion of the submandibular gland and duct.

The parapharyngeal space is bordered by the masticator and parotid spaces laterally, the carotid sheath posteriorly, and the submandibular space inferiorly. The medial border is pharyngeal mucosal surface, and it extends superiorly to the skull base. This space contains mostly fat as well as vascular structures such as the internal maxillary artery and descending pharyngeal artery. There are also lymph nodes and minor salivary glands.

(3) Infrahyoid Neck

The anterior visceral space extends from the thyroid cartilage superiorly to the superior mediastinum at the level of the 4th thoracic vertebrae. Anteriorly, it is limited by the strap muscles and visceral fascia.

(4) Length of the Neck

The retropharyngeal space lies between the visceral division of the middle layer of the deep cervical fascia and the deep layer of the cervical fascia. It is posterior to the hypopharynx and the esophagus, is medial to the carotid sheath, and extends inferiorly into mediastinum as far as the third thoracic vertebral body. The retropharyngeal space consists of loose connective tissue. The retropharyngeal space is divided by the the alar prevertebral fascia in both the front and rear ends into two parts: the anterior and posterior. The front area is called retropharyngeal space, while the rear area is called the "danger space". The alar parts of the prevertebral fascia extend along the cranial base and the cervical vertebrae, bordering the buccopharyngeal mucous membrane at the base (White, 1985; Haug et al., 1990; Chow, 1992; Hasegawa et al., 2007).

The prevertebral space is located behind the prevertebral layer of the deep cervical fascia. It contains the prevertebral and paraspinal muscles, vertebral bodies, disk spaces, and the vertebral artery and veins, and extends inferiorly along the spine to the coccyx.

DEEP NECK INFECTIONS

Deep neck infections are serious diseases that involve several spaces in the neck. Deep neck infections can arise from various neck regions, including teeth, salivary glands, the nasal cavity, paranasal sinuses, pharynx, and adenotonsillar tissues. The teeth are the most common primary site, followed by tonsils (Har-EL et al., 1997; Sethi et al, 1994; Bahu et al, 2001; Parhiscar et al, 2001; Sakaguchi et al, 1997; Virolainen et al., 1979; Lin et al., 2001; Levitt, 1971; Estrera et al., 1983; Furst et al., 2001; Georgalas et al., 2002; Johnson et al., 1976; Smith et al., 2003; Suehara et al., 2008). A deep neck abscess often starts as an isolated area of cellulitis in the soft tissues adjacent to the source of the infection (Stalfors et al., 2004; Brook et al., 2004). Since the fascial layers of the neck and the body's natural defense mechanisms help to prevent further spread of infection, widespread progression is not typically seen (Kim et al., 1997). However, if the infection is not adequately treated, it may develop into a purulent fluid collection (Daramola et al., 2009). The abscess may track along fascial planes deeper into the neck and potentially extend into the mediastinum (Huang et al., 2004; Bottin et al., 2003; Brook, 2004; Kim et al., 1997). The common symptoms of deep neck infections are neck pain, neck swelling, fever, sore throat, trismus, and odynophagia. Additional signs and symptoms include otalgia, dysphagia, oral swelling, and dyspnea (Daramola et al., 2009). However, present signs and symptoms vary and are dependent on the time at which a patient seeks medical attention.

Early studies of the bacteriology of deep neck infections have pointed out three microorganisms: S*taphylococcus aureus, Streptococcus pyogenes,* and anaerobic bacteria

(Tom et al., 1988; Barlett et al., 1976). Nowadays, mixed infections with both aerobic and anaerobic bacteria has become the rule (Har-El et al., 1997; Wills et al., 1981). Anaerobic bacteria, such as Fusobacteria species, and anaerobic streptococci (Peptostreptococci species), comprise 90% of bacteria by weight in the gingival crevice (Cummings, 2005). These anaerobic bacteria are often involved in deep neck infections. Streptococci are reportedly the organisms most commonly cultured from deep neck abscesses (Dodds et al., 1988; Thompson et al., 1988; Tom et al., 1988; Ungkanont et al., 1995).

Life-threatening complications include: descending mediastinitis, septic shock, upper airway obstruction, jugular vein thrombosis, and venous septic embolus (Beck et al., 1984). Descending necrotizing mediastinitis is the most feared complication; it results from retropharyngeal extension of the infection into the posterior mediastinum. Pleural and pericardic effusion may accompany this condition, frequently leading to cardiac tamponade. If septic shock occurs, it is reportedly associated with a 40-50% mortality rate (Chen et al., 2000).

DIAGNOSIS

History and Physical Examination

Evaluation of a patient with suspected deep neck infection usually starts with taking history and a physical examination. A detailed history should be taken from patients in whom deep neck space infection is suspected. Eliciting a history of the following is important:

- Pain (neck pain, sore throat)
- Recent dental procedures
- Upper respiratory tract infections
- Neck or oral cavity trauma
- Dyspnea
- Dysphagia
- Immunosuppression or immunocompromised status
- Rate of onset
- Duration of symptoms

Physical examination should focus on determining the location of the originating infection, the deep neck spaces involved, and any potential functional compromise or complications that may be developing. Specifically, a comprehensive head and neck examination should include special attention to teeth, tonsils (forcuses of the original infection), and obstructions of the airway. Neck pain caused by deep neck infections often involve fever, swelling of neck lymph nodes, and warmth and the redness of the neck. It is important for the clinician to suspect the presence of deep neck infections when neck pain is accompanied by such symptoms.

Laboratory Studies

Tests, including the following, may be useful in the workup of a patient in whom a deep neck space infection is suspected:

- Blood chemistries
- Complete blood cell count
- Blood cultures
- Abscess cultures with Gram stains

Imaging Studies

Imaging studies are essential for adequately evaluating patients with deep neck infections. Computed tomography (CT) scans are a mainstay of imaging studies of deep neck infections. Radiography became of limited value. However, some radiographical studies afford useful information to evaluate deep neck infections, if adequately employed.

Lateral neck radiography can image retropharyngeal soft tissues in the posterior wall of the hypopharynx to assess the retropharyngeal and pretracheal space. Dental radiographs, such as a Panorex oral view may also indicate where a dental infection is suspected. Particular attention should be given to the second and third mandibular molars because the apices of these teeth extend below the mylohyoid line, giving them access to the submandibular space (Cummings, 2005). Chest radiography (and/or CT scan) is indicated for all patients with deep neck infections to evaluate the severe complications, such as mediastinitis and pleural effusion.

Ultrasonography

High-resolution ultrasound has the advantages of being portable and not being ionizing radiation. It is therefore very useful in many departments. However, the reliability of the finding is operator dependent, and few studies support its use in diagnosis (Cummings, 2005). Ultrasounds do not reveal anatomic details but can help distinguish between phlegmon and abscesses, give information about the condition of surrounding vessels, and guide fine-needle aspiration (FNA) attempts.

CT Scanning

CT scans are fast, relatively inexpensive, and fairly widely available today. CT scans with contrast are the gold standard in the evaluation of deep neck infections. CT scans indicate the location, boundaries, and relation of infection to surrounding neurovascular structures. Findings that indicate a deep neck infection include a mass with an air-fluid interface or a cystic or multiloculated appearance, and edema, or contrast ("ring") enhancement of tissue surrounding mass (Holt et al., 1982). It has been shown to have a sensitivity ranging from 95 to 100 percent in identifying and characterizing deep neck infections (Bottin et al., 2003; Nagy et al., 1999). CT is instrumental in distinguishing superficial cellulites from abscess, in the localization of abscess, in the identification of airway deviation, and the involvement of the carotid sheath or major blood vessels (Stalfors et al., 2004; Kim et al., 1997; Brook, 2007; Nagy et al., 1999). CT scanning identifies specific problems such as tracheal compression, mediastinal spread, and internal jugular vein thrombosis. It is recommendable to extend the computed tomography scan from the neck to the mediastinum, in order to evaluate the spread of the infection in some situations, such as when neck swelling is observed to reach the suprasternal notch (Crespo et al., 2004).

Magnetic Resonance Imaging (MRI)

MRI offers better resolution of soft tissues, superior imaging of blood vessels, and no interference by dental findings. However, because of longer acquisition time and higher cost as compared with CT scanning, MRI may not be the initial modality of choice.

Management

Airway Management
Patients with deep neck infections may die as a result of airway management mishaps. Ensuring a secure airway is the first priority in the management of a deep neck infection. Therefore, it should always be considered if intubation or tracheotomy is necessary. Tissue edema and immobility, a distorted airway, and copious secretions are common in patients with deep neck infections, and contribute to the difficulty of establishing an airway. Thus, it is critical to make an adequate clinical judgment concerning timing and the method for airway intervention (Ovassapian et al., 2004). Ovassapian et al. (2004) reported fiberoptic intubation using topical anesthesia as the first choice for airway control in adult patients with deep neck infections. Tracheostomy under local anesthesia is a good choice if an attempt at intubation has failed, or if the clinician is not skilled with awake fiberoptic intubation (Ovassapion et al., 2004).

Antibiotic Treatment
Superficial infections, such as cellulites and, sometimes, even abscesses, can be managed with antibiotics alone (Plaza et al., 2001; Nagy et al., 1997). Empiric antibiotic coverage for deep neck infections must consider aerobic and anaerobic pathogens that synthesize beta-lactamase (Bottin et al., 2003; Brook, 2004; Brook, 2007; Rega et al., 2006). Second or third generation cephalosporin drugs and Clindamycin are effective. Alternatively, a penicillin and beta-lactamase inhibitor combination such as ampicillin-sulbactam also provides adequate coverage (Bottin et al., 2003; Rega et al., 2006). The possibility of a gram negative facultative anaerobe found in the oral cavity makes it reasonable to add ciprofloxacin or an aminoglycoside (Cummings, 2005). Antibiotic drugs may be changed by culture results. It is important to recognize that it is easier to manage with antibiotics alone as deep neck infections are treated in the earlier stages of the disease.

Surgical Management

Surgical drainage plays one of the leading roles in the treatment of deep neck infection. Surgical drainage is indicated for most deep abscesses, especially when there is a comprised airway, sepsis syndrome, or no response to antibiotic treatment within 48 hours (Gidley et al., 1997).

A large incision permits expansion of tissue, thereby reducing compartment pressure, and this may be critical in preventing extension of the infection from one space to adjacent spaces. This also allows better tissue oxygenation, with reduction of the anaerobic flora. The surgical approach can also assure upper airway patency in cases of actual or imminent upper respiratory distress (Crespo et al., 2004) in addition to debridement of necrotic tissue.

Deep Neck Infections Causing Neck Pain

Deep infections usually cause neck, throat, or facial pain. Deep neck infections, which seem to be important for differential diagnosis of neck pain, are described below.

Retropharyngeal Abscess

Retropharyngeal abscess is often associated with the severe inflammation of the retropharyngeal lymph nodes located in the retropharyngeal abscess after acute pharyngitis. Retropharyngeal abscess is predominantly an infection in childhood, partly because the retropharyngeal space is fairly open during childhood and becomes involuted with age, shrinking back after the age of 3 (Hasegawa et al., 2008). Sharma et al. (1998) reported that 90% of such cases have occurred in children below age 6. Nowadays, with the advancement of antibiotics, their incidence and severity have decreased significantly (Chen et al., 1998; Wang et al., 2003; Parhiscar et al., 2001). However, retropharyngeal abscess is observed with increasing frequency in adults (Hasegawa et al., 2008). Several reports have demonstrated that adult cases of retropharyngeal abscess are sometimes accompanied by spinal tuberculosis. Tuberculosis of the spine has a predilection for the middle and lower thoracic spine. Cervical tuberculous vertebral osteomyelitis is unusual, and tuberculosis reportedly affects the cervical vertebrae in approximately 0.03% of all cases (Wurtz et al., 1993). Retropharyngeal abscess causes severe neck pain, fever, and stiffness of the neck. When diagnosing retropharyngeal abscess, it is important for clinical management to determine whether it is a result of a pharyngeal infection or a result of spreading from a posterior infection, such as cervical osteomyelitis (Attia et al., 2004). Retropharyngeal abscess sometimes causes meningism and headache.

Ludwig's Angina

Ludwig's angina, a rapidly progressive cellulitis of the floor of the mouth, involves the submandibular, submaxillary, and sublingual spaces. Patients have severe neck pain, swelling, and elevation of the tongue, fever, neck swelling, and dysphagia. The most common cause of Ludwig's angina is an odontogenic infection, from one or more grossly decayed, infected tooth, and is usually a result of native oral streptococci or a mixed aerobic-anaerobic oral flora (Abramowicz et al., 2006). Additional possible etiological factors include sialadenitis, compound mandibular fractures, or puncture wounds of the floor of the mouth

(Abramowicz et al., 2006). The most feared complication is airway obstruction due to elevation and posterior displacement of the tongue (Duprey et al., 2010). It is important to recognize Ludwig's angina in the earlier stages of the disease to prevent airway obstruction.

Lemierre's Syndrome

Lemierre's syndrome is septic thrombophlebitis of the internal jugular vein, usually secondary to acute head and neck infections, and frequently complicated by metastasis infections, such as pulmonary emboli, septic arthritis, paravertebral abscess, and skin infections (Lemierre, 1936). This disorder develops primarily in healthy young adults. Initial symptoms are neck pain, fever, tenderness, or swelling of the lateral side of the neck or trismus. Anaerobic organisms lead to the development of septic thrombophlebitis of the internal jugular vein. Septicemia may follow about three to 10 days after the neck thrombophlebitis. *Fusobacterium necrophorum*, an anaerobic organism, is the main causative organism of Lemierre's syndrome (Repanos et al., 2006; Hoenhon et al., 2002; Karkos et al., 2004). Broad-spectrum antibiotics covering the anaerobic organism and debridement of the primary infectious lesions are the treatments of choice for Lemierre's syndrome (Karkos et al., 2004; Brown et al., 2007). The duration of treatment by antibiotic therapy is often lengthy, and the mean duration of the therapy reported in the related literature is 6 weeks, with a range from 2 to 14 weeks (Alvarez et al., 1995). The role of anticoagulants is also controversial in therapy for Lemierre's syndrome, although advocates of systemic anticoagulation cite the potential for faster resolution of the thrombophlebitis and bacteremia, limiting the development of new metastatic foci (Goldhagen et al., 1988; Lustig et al., 1995). The possibility of Lemierre's syndrome should thus be considered in those with neck pain, swelling of the lateral side of the neck, and with deep neck infections. A clinical suspicion of Lemierre's syndrome seems to be essential to make an accurate diagnosis during the early stage of the disease and archive a successful outcome (Nakayama et al., 2010).

CONCLUSION

Numerous conditions cause neck pain. Deep neck infections, albeit relatively rare, may also induce neck pain. Fascia in the neck consists of the deep neck spaces. Several infections, such as odontogenic, nasal/paranasal, parotid, pharyngeal, and vertebral infections, may spread to these spaces. The marked neck pain and inflammatory laboratory data suggests the presence of deep neck infections. CT scans with contrast enhancement are diagnostic, and MRIs are also helpful for the diagnosis of abscess and cellulitis. Deep neck infections may result in fatal complications including airway obstruction. Early diagnosis and interventions with appropriate antibiotics and airway managements, if necessary, are important for their proper management.

REFERENCES

Abramowicz S, Abramowicz JS, Dolwick MF. Severe Life Threatening Maxillofacial Infection in Pregnancy Presented as Ludwig's Angina. *Infect Dis Obstet Gynecol*. 2006; 2006: 51931.

Alvarez A, Schreider JR. Lemierre`s syndrome in adolescent children: Anaerobic sepsis with internal jugular vein thrombophlebitis following pharyngitis. *Pediatrics.* 1995; 96: 354-359.

Attia M, Harnof S, Knoller N, Shacked I, Zibly Z, Bedrin L, Regev-Yochay G. Cervical Pott's disease presenting as a retropharyngeal abscess. *Isr Med Assoc J.* 2004; 6: 438-439.

Bahu SJ, Shibuya TY, Meleca RJ, Mathog RH, Yoo GH, Stachler RJ, Tyburski JG. Craniocervical necrotizing fasciitis: an 11-year experience. *Otolaryngol Head Neck Surg.* 2001; 125: 245-252.

Barker J, Winer-Muram HT, Grey S. Lemierre syndrome. *Southern Med. J.* 1996; 89: 1021-1023.

Barlett JG, Froggatt JW: Antibiotic resistance. *Arch Otolaryngol Head Neck Surg.* 1995; 121: 392-396.

Barlett JG, Gorbach SL. Anaerobic infections of the head and neck. *Otolaryngol clin North Am.* 1976; 9: 655-678.

Beck HJ, Salassa JR, McCaffrey TV, Hermans PE. Life-threatening soft-tissue infections of the neck. *Laryngoscope.* 1984; 94: 354-362.

Bottin R, Marioni G, Rinaldi R, Boninsegna M, Salvadori L, Staffieri A. Deep neck infection: a present-day complication. A retrospective review of 83 cases (1998-2001). *Eur. Arch Otorhinolaryngol.* 2003; 260: 576-579.

Brook I. Microbiology and management of peritonsillar, retropharyngeal, and parapharyngeal abscesses. *J. Oral Maxillofac Surg.* 2004; 62: 1545-1550.

Brook I. The role of anaerobic bacteria in upper respiratory tract and other head and neck infections.*Curr. Infect. Dis. Rep.* 2007; 9: 208-217.

Brown M, Wallwork B. Lemierre`s-the sinister sore throat. *J. Laryngol. Otol.* 2007; 121: 692-694.

Chen MK, Wen YS, Chang CC, Huang MT, Hsiao HC. Predisposing factors of life-threatening deep neck infection: logistic regression analysis of 214 cases. *J. Otolaryngol.* 1998; 27: 141-144.

Chen MK, Wen YS, Chang CC, Lee HS, Huang MT, Hsiao HC. Deep neck infections in diabetic patients. *Am. J. Otolaryngol.* 2000; 21: 169-173.

Chow AW: Life-threatening infections of the head and neck. Clin Infect Dis. 1992; 14: 991-1002.

Coonan KM, Kaplan EL: In vitro susceptibility of recent North American group A streptococcal isolates to eleven oral antibiotics. *Pediatr. Infect Dis J.* 1994; 13: 630-635.

Craig FW, Schunk JE: Retropharyngeal abscess in children: clinical presentation, utility of imaging, and current management. *Pediatrics.* 2003; 111: 1394-1398.

Crespo AN, Chone CT, Fonseca AS, Montenegro MC, Pereira R, Milani JA. Clinical versus computed tomography evaluation in the diagnosis and management of deep neck infection. *Sao Paulo Med J.* 2004; 122: 259-263.

Cummings CW, Flint PW, Haughey BH, et al. *Otolaryngology: Head and Neck Surgery.* 4th ed. St Louis, Mo; Mosby; 2005: 4365-4367.

Daramola OO, Flanagan CE, Maisel RH, Odland RM. Diagnosis and treatment of deep neck space abscesses. *Otolaryngol Head Neck Surg.* 2009; 141: 123-130.

Dodds B, Maniglia AJ. Peritonsillar and neck abscesses in the pediatric age group. *Laryngoscope.* 1988; 98: 956-959.

Duprey K, Rose J, Fromm C. Ludwig's angina. *Int. J. Emerg. Med.* 2010; 3: 201-202.

Estrera AS, Landay MJ, Grisham JM, Sinn DP, Platt MR. Descending necrotizing mediastinitis.*Surg. Gynecol. Obstet.* 1983; 157: 545-552.

Furst IM, Ersil P, Caminiti M. A rare complication of tooth abscess--Ludwig's angina and mediastinitis. *J. Can Dent Assoc.* 2001; 67: 324-327.

Georgalas C, Kanagalingam J, Zainal A, Ahmed H, Singh A, Patel KS. The association between periodontal disease and peritonsillar infection: a prospective study. *Otolaryngol Head Neck Surg.* 2002; 126: 91-94.

Gidley PW, Ghorayeb BY, Stiernberg CM. Contemporary management of deep neck space infections. *Otolaryngol. Head Neck Surg.* 1997; 116: 16-22.

Goldhagen J, Alford BA, Prewitt LH, Thompson L, Hostetter MK. Suppurative thrombophlebitis of the internal jugular vein: report three cases and reveiw of the pediatric literature. *Pediatr. Infect. Dis J.* 1988; 7: 410-414

Har-El G, Aroesty JH, Shaha A, Lucente FE. Changing trends in deep neck abscess. A retrospective study of 110 patients. *Oral Surg. Oral Med Oral Pathol.* 1994; 77: 446-450.

Hasegawa J, Tateda M, Hidaka H, Sagai S, Nakanome A, Katagiri K, Seki M, Katori Y, Kobayashi T. Retropharyngeal abscess complicated with torticollis: case report and review of the literature. *Tohoku J. Exp. Med.* 2007; 213: 99-104.

Haug RH, Picard U, Indresano AT. Diagnosis and treatment of the retropharyngeal abscess in adults. *Br. J. Oral Maxillofac Surg.* 1990; 28: 34-38.

Hoenhon S., Dominguez T.E. Lemierre's syndrome An usual cause of sepsis and abdominal pain. *Crit. Care Med.* 2002; 30: 1644-1647.

Holt GR, McManus K, Newman RK, Potter JL, Tinsley PP. Computed tomography in the diagnosis of deep-neck infections. *Arch. Otolaryngol.* 1982; 108: 693-696.

Huang TT, Liu TC, Chen PR, Tseng FY, Yeh TH, Chen YS. Deep neck infection: analysis of 185 cases. *Head Neck.* 2004; 26: 854-860.

Johnson JT, Tucker HM. Recognizing and treating deep neck infection. *Postgrad Med.* 1976; 59: 95-100.

Karkos PD, Karkanevatos A, Panagea S, Dingle A, Davies JE. Lemierre's syndrome: how a sore throat can end in disaster. *Eur. J. Emerg. Med.* 2004; 11: 228-230.

Kim HJ, Park ED, Kim JH, Hwang EG, Chung SH. Odontogenic versus nonodontogenic deep neck space infections: CT manifestations. *J. Comput. Assist Tomogr.* 1997; 21: 202-208.

Lemierre A. On certain septicemias due to anaerobic organisms. Lancet 1936; 1: 701-703.

Levitt GW. The surgical treatment of deep neck infections. *Laryngoscope.* 1971; 81: 403-411.

Lin C, Yeh FL, Lin JT, Ma H, Hwang CH, Shen BH, Fang RH. Necrotizing fasciitis of the head and neck: an analysis of 47 cases. *Plast Reconstr. Surg.* 2001; 107: 1684-1693.

Lustig LR, Cusick BC, Cheng SW, Lee KC. Lemierres syndrome: two cases posangial sepsis. *Otolaryngol Head Neck Surg.* 1995; 112: 767-772.

Nagy M, Pizzuto M, Backstrom J, Brodsky L. Deep neck infections in children: a new approach to diagnosis and treatment. *Laryngoscope.* 1997; 107: 1627-1634.

Ovassapian A, Tuncbilek M, Weitzel EK, Joshi CW. Airway management in adult patients with deep neck infections: a case series and review of the literature. *Anesth Analg.* 2005; 100: 585-589.

Parhiscar A, Har-El G. Deep neck abscess: a retrospective review of 210 cases. *Ann Otol Rhinol Laryngol.* 2001; 110: 1051-1054.

Plaza Mayor G, Martinez-San illan J, Martinez-Vidal A. Is conservative treatment of deep neck space infections appropriate? *Head Neck.* 2001; 23: 126-133.

Rega AJ, Aziz SR, Ziccardi VB. Microbiology and antibiotic sensitivities of head and neck space infections of odontogenic origin. *J. Oral Maxillofac. Surg.* 2006; 64: 1377-1380.

Repanos C, Chadha NK, Griffiths MV. Sigmoid sinus thrombosis secondary to Lemierre Syndrome. *Ear. Nose Throat J.* 2006; 85: 98-101.

Sakaguchi M, Sato S, Ishiyama T, Katsuno S, Taguchi K. Characterization and management of deep neck infections. *Int. J. Oral Maxillofac Surg.* 1997; 26: 131-134.

Sethi DS, Stanley RE. Deep neck abscesses--changing trends. *Laryngol Otol.* 1994; 108: 138-143.

Sharma HS, Kurl DN, Hamzah M. Retropharyngeal abscess: recent trends. *Auris Nasus Larynx.* 1998; 25: 403-406.

Smith L, Osborne R. Infections of the head and neck. *Top Emerg Med.* 2003; 25: 106-116.

Stalfors J, Adielsson A, Ebenfelt A, Nethander G, Westin T. Deep neck space infections remain a surgical challenge. A study of 72 patients. *Acta Otolaryngol.* 2004; 124: 1191-1196.

Suehara AB, Gonçalves AJ, Alcadipani FA, Kavabata NK, Menezes MB. Deep neck infections: analysis of 80 cases. *Braz. J. Otorhinolaryngol.* 2008; 74: 253-259.

Tom MB, Rice DH. Presentation and management of neck abscess: a retrospective analysis. *Laryngoscope.* 1988; 98: 877-880.

Thompson JW, Cohen SR, Reddix P. Retropharyngeal abscess in children: a retrospective and historical analysis. *Int. J. Pediatr. Otorhinolaryngol.* 1988; 15: 179-184.

Ungkanont K, Yellon RF, Weissman JL, Casselbrant ML, González-Valdepeña H, Bluestone CD. Head and neck space infections in infants and children. *Otolaryngol. Head Neck Surg.* 1995; 112: 375-382.

Virolainen E, Haapaniemi J, Aitasalo K, Suonpää J. Deep neck infections. Int J Oral Surg. 1979; 8: 407-411.

Wang LF, Kuo WR, Tsai SM, Huang KJ. Characterizations of life-threatening deep cervical space infections: a review of one hundred ninety-six cases. *Am. J. Otolaryngol.* 2003; 24: 111-117.

White B. Deep neck infections and respiratory distress in children. *Ear. Nose Throat J.* 1985; 64: 30-38.

Wills PI, Vernon RP. Complications of space infections of the head and neck. *Laryngoscope.* 1981; 91: 1129-1136.

Wurtz R, Quader Z, Simon D, Langer B. Cervical tuberculous vertebral osteomyelitis: case report and discussion of the literature. *Clin. Infect Dis.* 1993; 16: 806-808.

In: Neck Pain: Causes, Diagnosis and Management
Editor: Gregorio Lombardi

ISBN 978-1-61470-363-1
© 2012 Nova Science Publishers, Inc.

Chapter 5

EXPERIMENTAL NECK MUSCLES PAIN, STANDING BALANCE AND PROPRIOCEPTION

Nicolas Vuillerme*[1], Petra Hlavackova[1], Antoine Pradels[2], Céline Franco[3] and Jacques Vaillant[4]

[1]FRE 3405, AGIM (AGeing Imaging Modeling), Grenoble, France
[2]FRE 3405, AGIM (AGeing Imaging Modeling), Grenoble, France and Centre de Podologie de l'Estacade, France
[3]FRE 3405, AGIM (AGeing Imaging Modeling), Grenoble, France and IDS, Montceau les Mines
[4]FRE 3405, AGIM (AGeing Imaging Modeling), Grenoble, France and School of Physiotherapy, Grenoble University Hospital Grenoble, France

ABSTRACT

In this study, we used an experimental pain model to provide painful stimulation on the neck muscles to assess the effect of neck muscles pain on the control of unperturbed bipedal posture and on neck proprioception. Sixteen young asymptomatic adults voluntarily participated in two separate experiments.

In experiment 1, participants (n=8) were asked to stand upright, as still as possible, in three experimental conditions : (1) a no pain condition, (2) a condition when a painful stimulation was applied to the neck muscles and (3) a condition in which painful stimulation was applied to another body part, the palms of both hands. The centre of foot pressure displacements were recorded using a on a force platform. Results showed that, for the same perceived intensity of the pain, the painful stimulation applied to the neck muscles increased centre of foot pressure displacements, whereas the painful stimulation applied to the palms of both hands did not. Results of experiment 1 demonstrated the deleterious effect of experimentally-induced pain on the neck muscles on unperturbed bipedal postural control and suggest that the painful stimulation affects the postural

---

* Address for correspondence: Nicolas Vuillerme, FRE 3405, AGIM (AGeing Imaging Modeling), CNRS-UJF-EPHE, Grenoble, France. Faculty of Medicine. 38706 La Tronche Cedex. France. Email: nicolas.vuillerme@agim.eu

control mechanisms through sensori-motor mechanisms rather than through cognitive resources related to the perception of pain.

Experiment 2 was specifically designed to address this issue by assessing the effect of on experimental neck muscles pain on cervical joint position sense. To this end, participants (n=8) were asked to execute a clinical test usually employed to the cervical joint position sense, the Cervicocephalic Repositioning Test (CRT) CRT to Neutral Head Position (NHP). In this assessment, a blindfolded subject seated on a chair with the head in NHP is asked to relocate the head on the trunk, as accurately as possible, after full active cervical rotation to the left and right sides, and absolute and variable errors were used to assess accuracy and consistency of the repositioning, respectively. The CRT to NHP was performed in two experimental conditions presented in Experiment 1: (1) a no pain condition, (2) a condition when a painful stimulation was applied to the neck muscles. Results showed that the painful stimulation applied to the neck muscles induced less accurate and less consistent repositioning performances. Results of experiment 2 demonstrated the deleterious effect of experimentally-induced pain on the neck muscles on cervical joint position sense, assessed through the CRT to the NHP.

Taken together, results of Experiments 1 and 2 suggest experimental neck muscle pain affected control of unperturbed bipedal posture via altered proprioceptive inflow.

1. INTRODUCTION

Although impaired balance control during quiet standing (e.g., [Alund et al., 1993; Dehner et al., 2008; Karlberg et al., 1995; Madeleine et al., 2004; Michaelson et al., 2003; Persson et al., 1996; Poole et al., 2008; Treleaven et al., 2005]) and deteriorated neck proprioceptive acuity (e.g., [Cheng et al., 2010; Heikkila and Astrom, 1996; Kristjansson et al., 2003; Pinsault et al., 2008; Revel et al., 1991; Treleaven et al., 2003]) have repeatedly been reported in persons suffering from neck pain in patients suffering from chronic neck pain of both traumatic and non-traumatic aetiologies, a better understanding of the effect of neck muscles pain on unperturbed postural control is needed. Indeed, causality cannot be determined in clinical cross-sectional studies since any confounding effect of neck pain with age and/or with an underlying pathology and/or adaptive adjustments of motor control strategies cannot be a priori excluded. Thus, to isolate systematically the influence of neck muscle pain, we previously used an experimental pain model to provide painful stimulation on the neck muscles to assess the effect of neck muscles pain *per se* on the control of unperturbed bipedal posture [Vuillerme and Pinsault, 2009]. Indeed, this paradigm does present the advantage of standardizing the origin, the locus, the intensity and the duration of muscle pain [Svensson and Arendt-Nielsen, 1995]. Along these lines, young asymptomatic adults were asked to stand upright as still as possible on a force platform with their eyes closed in two conditions of No pain and Pain of the neck muscles elicited by experimental painful electrical stimulation. Analysis of centre of foot pressure (CoP) displacements showed that experimental neck muscle pain deteriorated the control of unperturbed bipedal posture. It has been suggested that the painful stimulation affected the postural control mechanisms through sensori-motor mechanisms rather than through cognitive resources related to the perception of pain [Vuillerme and Pinsault, 2009]. The present experiment was thus designed to investigate this issue in more depth. Two separated experiment were conducted on young asymptomatic adults. The purpose of Experiment 1 was to assess the effect of experimental neck muscle pain on postural control during unperturbed stance by comparing centre of foot pressure (CoP) displacements recorded in a condition when a painful stimulation was applied to the neck muscles with CoP displacements during a no pain condition and also with CoP displacements recorded in a condition in which painful stimulation was applied to another body part [Corbeil et al., 2004; Pradels et al., 2011]: the palms of both hands. The purpose of Experiment 2 was to assess the effect of of experimental neck muscle pain on cervical joint position sense.

2. METHODS

2.1. Participants

A total of sixteen participants took part in this study. Eight young asymptomatic male adults (mean age= 21.1 (SD 1.1) years; mean body weight= 70.1 (SD 4.2) kg; mean height= 176.4 (SD 6.3) cm) voluntarily in Experiment 1. Eight young asymptomatic male adults (mean age= 22.4 (SD 1.6) years; mean body weight= 72.1 (SD 4.4) kg; mean height= 178.0 (SD 5.7) cm) voluntarily participated in Experiment 2. None of them had participated in Experiment 2.

Criteria for selection and inclusion were: male; aged 20-30 years. Exclusion criteria were: sagittal and/or coronal alignment of the neck impairment, history of motor problem, neck pain, neurological disease or vestibular impairment.

Participants were familiarized with the experimental procedure and apparatus and they gave their informed consent to the experimental procedure as required by the Helsinki declaration (1964) and the local Ethics Committee, and were naive as to the purpose of the experiment.

2.2. Experimental Procedures

Two separate experiments were conducted.

2.2.1. Experiment 1: Postural Control during Unperturbed Stance

Experimental Task

Participants stood barefoot on a force platform (Dynatronic, France; sampling frequency: 40Hz) in a natural but standardised position (feet abducted at 30°, heels 3-cm apart), their arms hanging loosely by their sides and their eyes closed.

They were asked to stand as still as possible [Zok et al., 2008] during three experimental conditions: No-pain, Neck-pain and Palmar-pain. The No pain condition served as a control condition. In the two Pain conditions, painful electrical stimulations were applied either to the muscle belly of the pars descendents of Trapezius muscles of both sides (Neck-pain condition) [Vuillerme and Pinsault, 2009], or the dorsum of the first and second metacarpal heads of both hands (Palmar-pain condition). This electrical stimulation created a focal cutaneous painful stimulus with very limited current spread. The amplitude used for the stimulation was determined when the participants quoted the perceived pain intensity of the stimulation equal to 7 on a 0–10 visual analog scale [Price et al., 1983].

Three 25.6-s trials for each experimental condition were performed. The order of presentation of the three experimental conditions was randomized over the participants. No feedback was given to the subjects about their actual postural performance.

Pain Intensity Assessment

At the end of each trial, subjects were asked to rate their perception of the intensity of the pain induced by the stimulation by indicating the level on a 10-cm visual analog scale where 0-cm indicated "no pain" and 10-cm "intolerable pain". Use of visual analog scales to measure experimental pain has been validated [Price et al., 1983].

Balance Assessment

Two dependent variables were used to describe the participants' postural behaviour:

1) the surface area (mm²) covered by the trajectory of the CoP providing a measure of the CoP spatial variability,
2) the mean velocity of the CoP displacements (mm/s) (the total distance covered by the CoP divided by the duration of the sampled period), constituting a good index of the amount of activity required to maintain stability [Geurts et al., 1993; Maki et al., 1990].

Note that results of a recent study have established the "excellent" test-retest reliability of these dependant variables [Pinsault and Vuillerme, 2009].

Statistical Analysis

Data obtained in the No-pain, Neck-pain and Palmar-pain conditions were compared using t tests. Level of significance was set at 0.05.

2.2.2. Experiment 2: Cervical Joint Position Sense

The purpose of the first experiment was to assess the effect of experimental neck muscle pain on cervical joint position sense.

Experimental Task

Participants were asked to perform the CRT to NHP [Revel et al., 1991]. Participants were seated on a chair with a backrest at three meters from a white wall filmed during all the experiment, with the head in a neutral position. They were asked to relocate the head on the trunk to the NHP with a maximum of precision, without speed instruction, after active head movement performed in the horizontal plane within comfortable limits. Participants had a laser pointer attached on the head and a handheld button to switch it on to materialize their NHP before and after head relocation. All laser impacts, characterizing head positions before and after repositioning, were recorded by a camera. A software program was developed to automatically determine head repositioning errors corresponding to the difference, in degrees, between laser impacts coordinates before and after head repositioning.

This proprioceptive task was executed in two experimental conditions: No-pain and Neck-pain. As for the Experiment 1, the No-pain condition served as a control condition, whereas, in the Neck-pain condition, painful electrical stimulations for which the amplitude determined when the participants quoted their perceived pain intensity of the stimulation equal to 7 on a 0–10 visual analog scale [Price et al., 1983], were applied to the muscle belly of the pars descendents of Trapezius muscles of both sides.

For each experimental condition, participants executed ten trials after a right head rotation (RR) and ten after a left head rotation (LR). The order of presentation of the two experimental conditions was randomized over the participants. No feedback was given to the subjects about their actual proprioceptive performance.

Pain Intensity Assessment

At the end of each trial, subjects were asked to rate their perception of the intensity of the pain induced by the stimulation by indicating the level on a 10-cm visual analog scale where 0-cm indicated "no pain" and 10-cm "intolerable pain".

Proprioceptive Assessment

Two dependent variables were used to assess proprioceptive performances [Schmidt, 1988]:

1) the absolute error (AE in degrees) as a measure of the overall accuracy of the repositioning; and
2) the variable error (VE in degrees) as a measure of the variability of the repositioning.

Note that results of a recent study using have established the "excellent" test-retest reliability of these dependant variables [Pinsault et al., 2008].

Statistical Analysis

Paired sample t-tests revealed no differences regarding mean AE and VE values between right and left rotation sides ($Ps > 0.05$). AE and VE obtained in the No-pain and Neck-pain conditions were compared using t tests. Level of significance was set at 0.05.

3. RESULTS

3.1. Experiment 1: Postural Control during Unperturbed Stance

Perceived Pain Intensity Values

Analysis of the visual analog scores showed higher values of perceived pain intensity were observed in the Neck-pain and the Palmar-pain conditions relative to the No-pain condition (P<0.001). Furthermore, no statistical difference were observed between values of perceived pain intensity scores observed in the Neck-pain condition and those observed in the Palmar-pain condition (P>0.05).

Postural Parameters

Analysis of the CoP surface area showed that the Neck-pain condition yields a wider CoP surface area relative to the No-pain and the Palmar-pain conditions ($P<0.05$), whereas no statistical difference between the CoP surface area measured in the Palmar-pain and No-pain conditions was observed ($P>0.05$) (Figure 1).

Analysis of the CoP mean velocity showed that the Neck-pain condition yields a higher CoP mean velocity relative to the No-pain and the Palmar-pain conditions ($P<0.001$), whereas no statistical difference between the CoP mean velocity measured in the Palmar-pain and No-pain conditions was observed ($P>0.05$) (Figure 2).

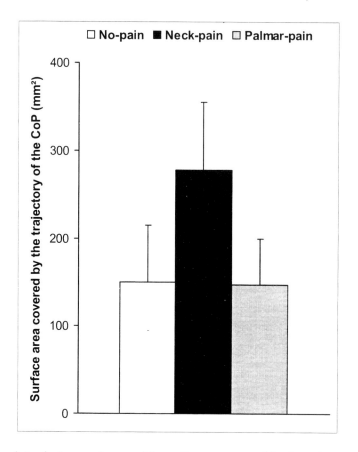

Figure 1. Mean and standard error of mean of the surface area covered by the trajectory of the centre of foot pressure (CoP) obtained in the three conditions of No-pain, Neck-pain and Palmar-pain. Each of the three experimental conditions is presented with a different symbol: No-pain (*white bars*), Neck-pain (*black bars*) and Palmar-pain (*grey bars*).

3.2. Experiment 2: Cervical Joint Position Sense

Perceived Pain Intensity Values

Analysis of the visual analog scores showed higher values of perceived pain intensity were observed in the Neck-pain and the Palmar-pain conditions relative to the No-pain condition ($P<0.001$).

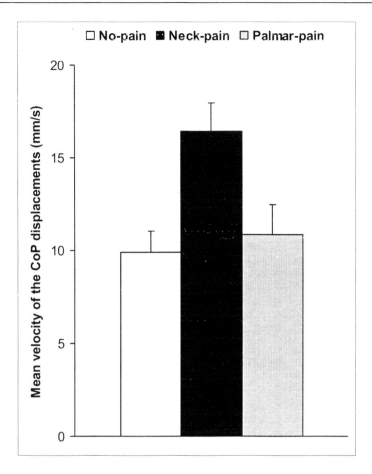

Figure 2. Mean and standard error of mean of the mean velocity of the centre of foot pressure (CoP) displacements obtained in the three conditions of No-pain, Neck-pain and Palmar-pain. Each of the three experimental conditions is presented with a different symbol: No-pain (*white bars*), Neck-pain (*black bars*) and Palmar-pain (*grey bars*).

Furthermore, no statistical difference were observed between values of perceived pain intensity scores observed in the Neck-pain condition and those observed in the Palmar-pain condition ($P>0.05$).

Proprioceptive Parameters

Analysis of the AE Showed higher values in the Neck-pain than No-pain condition ($P<0.001$; Figure 3).

Analysis of the VE also showed higher values in the Neck-pain than No-pain condition ($P<0.01$; Figure 4).

4. DISCUSSION

The purpose of the present study was to assess to assess the effect of experimental neck muscle pain on postural control during unperturbed stance and on neck proprioception.

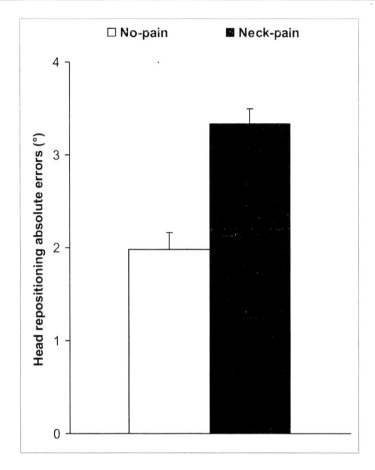

Figure 3. Mean and standard error of mean of the absolute errors obtained in the two conditions of No-pain and Neck-pain. Each of the two experimental conditions is presented with a different symbol: No-pain (*white bars*) and Neck-pain (*black bars*).

Sixteen young asymptomatic male adults voluntarily participated in the two separate experiments.

In experiment 1, participants (n=8) were asked to stand upright, as still as possible, in three experimental conditions : (1) a no pain condition, (2) a condition when a painful stimulation was applied to the neck muscles and (3) a condition in which painful stimulation was applied to another body part, the palms of both hands. The centre of foot pressure displacements were recorded using a force platform.

Before considering the effects on postural control during unperturbed stance, it is important to mention that the visual analogue scores clearly indicated that the electrical stimulations used in the Neck-pain and Palmar pain conditions were both painful and that in both conditions, the pain was similarly perceived as severe.

Analyses of the CoP displacements suggests that a painful stimulation applied to the neck muscles deteriorated postural control during unperturbed stance, as indicated by the increased surface area (Figure 1) and mean velocity (Figure 2) observed in the Neck-pain condition relative to both the No-pain and the Palmar-pain conditions.

Considering the functional significance of these CoP-based parameters (Geurts et al., 1993; Maki et al., 1990), these results suggest that the painful stimulation applied to the neck muscles degraded the effectiveness of the postural control system and increased the amount of postural regulatory activity required to control unperturbed bipedal posture a given posture. Conversely, analyses of the CoP displacements further showed no significant difference between the CoP displacements measured in the Palmar-pain condition and those measured in the No-pain condition.

Taken together, these results demonstrate that, for the same perceived intensity of the pain, the severe painful stimulation applied to the neck muscles degraded upright postural control, whereas the severe painful stimulation applied to the palms of both hands did not. Although the location of the painful stimulation was different, these results are in line with those previously reported by Corbeil et al. (2004) (dorsum of the first tarso-metatarsal joint of both feet and of the first and second metacarpal heads of both hands) and Pradels et al. (2011) (plantar surfaces of both feet and palms of both hands). These results hence suggest that experimentally-induced pain could affect postural control mechanisms through sensorimotor mechanisms rather than through cognitive resources related to the perception of pain [Eccleston and Crombez, 1999]. Without direct measures of the neck proprioceptive function, such proposal was speculative.

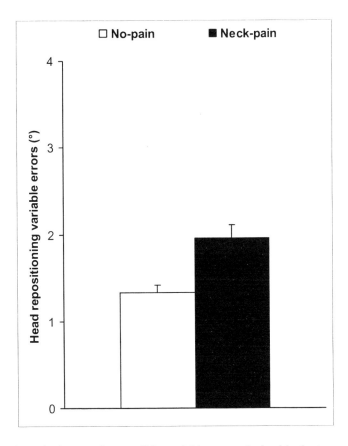

Figure 4. Mean and standard error of mean of the variable errors obtained in the two conditions of No-pain and Neck-pain. Each of the two experimental conditions is presented with a different symbol: No-pain (*white bars*) and Neck-pain (*black bars*).

Experiment 2 was hence specifically designed to address this issue by assessing the effect of on experimental neck muscles pain on cervical joint position sense. To this end, participants (n=8) were asked to execute a clinical test usually employed to the cervical joint position sense, the Cervicocephalic Repositioning Test (CRT) CRT to Neutral Head Position (NHP). In this assessment, a blindfolded subject seated on a chair with the head in NHP is asked to relocate the head on the trunk, as accurately as possible, after full active cervical rotation to the left and right sides, and absolute and variable errors were used to assess accuracy and consistency of the repositioning, respectively. The CRT to NHP was performed in two experimental conditions presented in Experiment 1: (1) a no pain condition, (2) a condition when a painful stimulation was applied to the neck muscles.

Before considering the effects on cervical joint position sense, it is important to mention that the visual analogue scores clearly indicated that the electrical stimulation used in the Neck-pain condition of Experiment 2 was painful.

Analysis of absolute errors (Figure 3) and variable errors Figure 4) showed that head repositioning performances were less accurate and less consistent in the Neck-pain relative to No-pain condition, respectively. On the whole, results of experiment 2 demonstrated the deleterious effect of experimentally-induced pain on the neck muscles on cervical joint position sense, assessed through the CRT to the NHP.

Taken together, results of Experiments 1 and 2 suggest experimental neck muscle pain affected control of unperturbed bipedal posture via altered proprioceptive inflow. At this point, however, a potential limitation of the present study pertains to the experimental design of this study. Experiment 1 and experiment 2 were performed with distinct groups of participants, so that there is no way of knowing whether the participants who degraded their cervical joint position sense would also degrade their postural control during unperturbed stance. Accordingly, a future experiment is our immediate plan to address this issue.

REFERENCES

Alund, M., Ledin, T., Odkvist, L., Larsson S.E. (1993) Dynamic posturography among patients with common neck disorders. A study of 15 cases with suspected cervical vertigo. *J. Vestib. Res*, 3, 383-389.

Cheng, C.H., Wang, J.L., Lin, J.J., Wang, S.F., Lin K.H. (2010) Position accuracy and electromyographic responses during head reposition in young adults with chronic neck pain. *J. Electromyogr Kinesiol*, 20, 1014-20.

Corbeil, P., Blouin, J.S., Teasdale N. (2004). Effects of intensity and locus of painful stimulation on postural stability. *Pain,* 108, 43-50.

Dehner, C., Heym., B., Maier, D., Sander, S., Arand, M., Elbel, M., Hartwig, E., Kramer, M. (2008) Postural control deficit in acute QTF grade II whiplash injuries. *Gait and Posture,* 28, 113-119.

Geurts, A.C.H., Nienhuis, B., Mulder, T.W. (1993) Intrasubject variability of selected force-platform parameters in the quantification of postural control. *Arch. Phys. Med. Rehabil*, 74, 1144-1150.

Heikkilä, H., Aström, P.G. (1996) Cervicocephalic kinesthetic sensibility in patients with whiplash injury. *Scand J. Rehabil. Med.,* 28, 133-138.

Karlberg, M., Persson, L., Magnusson M. (1995) Reduced postural control in patients with chronic cervicobrachial pain syndrome. *Gait and Posture*, 3, 241-249.

Kristjansson, E., Dall'Alba, P., Jull, G. (2003) A study of five cervicocephalic relocation tests in three different subject groups. *Clin. Rehabil*, 17, 768-774.

Madeleine, P., Prietzel, H., Svarrer, H., Arendt-Nielsen, L. (2004) Quantitative posturography in altered sensory conditions – A way to assess balance instability in patients with chronic whiplash injury. *Arch. Phys. Med. Rehabil*, 85, 432-438.

Maki, B., Holliday, P., Femie, G. (1990) Aging and postural control: a comparison of spontaneous- and induced-sway balance tests. *J. Am. Geriatr. Soc*, 38, 1-9.

Michaelson, P., Michaelson, M., Jaric, S., Latash, M.L., Sjolander, P., Djupsjobacka, M. (2003) Vertical posture and head stability in patients with chronic neck pain. *J. Rehabil Med*, 35, 229-235.

Persson, L., Karlberg, M., Magnusson, M. (1996) Effects of different treatments on postural performance in patients with cervical root compression. A randomized prospective study assessing the importance of the neck in postural control. *J. Vestib. Res*, 6, 439-453.

Pinsault, N, Fleury, A, Virone, G, Bouvier, B., Vaillant, J., Vuillerme, N. (2008) Test-retest reliability of cervicocephalic relocation test to the neutral head position. *Physiother Theory Pract*, 24, 380-391.

Pinsault, N., Vuillerme, N. (2009) Test-retest reliability of centre of foot pressure measures to assess postural control during unperturbed stance. *Med. Eng. Phys*, 31, 276-286.

Poole, E., Treleaven, J., Jull G. (2008) The influence of neck pain on balance and gait parameters in community-dwelling elders. *Man Ther*, 13, 317-324.

Pradels, A., Pradon, D., Vuillerme, N. (2011) Effects of experimentally-induced pain on the plantar soles on centre of foot pressure displacements during unperturbed upright stance. *Clinical Biomechanics*, 26, 424-428.

Price, D.D., McGrath, P.A., Rafii A. Buckingham B (1983) The validation of visual analogue scales as ratio scale measures for chronic and experimental pain. *Pain*, 17, 45-56.

Revel, M., Andre-Deshays, C., Minguet, M. (1991) Cervicocephalic kinesthetic sensibility in patients with cervical pain. *Arch. Phys. Med. Rehabil*, 72, 288-291.

Revel, M., Andre-Deshays, C., Minguet, M. (1991) Cervicocephalic kinesthetic sensibility in patients with cervical pain. *Arch. Phys Med. Rehabil*, 72, 288-291.

Schmidt, R. *Motor control and learning. A behavioral emphasis*. 2nd ed. Champaign: Human Kinetics Publishers Inc, 1988.

Treleaven, J., Jull, G., Sterling, M. (2003) Dizziness and unsteadiness following whiplash injury: characteristic features and relationship with cervical joint position error. *J. Rehab Med*, 35, 36-43.

Treleaven, J., Murison, R., Jull, G., LowChoy, N., Brauer, S. (2005) Is the method of signal analysis and test selection important for measuring standing balance in subjects with persistent whiplash? *Gait and Posture*, 21, 395-402.

Vuillerme, N., Pinsault, N. (2009) Experimental neck muscle pain impairs standing balance in humans. *Exp. Brain Res*, 192, 723-729.

Zok, M., Mazzà, C., Cappozzo, A. (2008) Should the instructions issued to the subject in traditional static posturography be standardised? *Med. Eng. Phys.*, 30, 913-916.

In: Neck Pain: Causes, Diagnosis and Management ISBN 978-1-61470-363-1
Editor: Gregorio Lombardi © 2012 Nova Science Publishers, Inc.

Chapter 6

PHARMACOLOGICAL INTERVENTION IN MANAGEMENT OF NECK PAIN DISORDERS: A REVIEW

Marwan S. M. Al-Nimer*

Pharmacology, College of Medicine,
Al-Mustansiriya University,
Baghdad, Iraq

ABSTRACT

The prevalence of neck pain disorders is increasing worldwide. Approximately 10% of adult have neck pain at any one time and less than 1% develop neurological deficit. The treatment of neck pain depends on its precise cause. It includes: rest, heat/ice application, traction, soft collar traction, physical therapy, transcutaneous electric nerve stimulation, surgical procedures and pharmacotherapy. The current pharmacological agents that used in management of neck pain include: non steroidal anti-inflammatory drugs, centrally acting analgesia, acetaminophen, muscle relaxants, topical painkillers and/or topical anesthesia, local steroids and/or local anesthetics injections and antimicrobials.

This review focuses on the concepts of pharmacotherapy of neck pain disorders in respect to the cause of neck pain, the nature of pain (acute, chronic, neuropathic or nociceptive), the mechanism of drug action, the practice of local injections with radiologist intervention, quality of life and the long term harmful effects including medicines abused. Also this review describes the beneficial effect of tumor necrosis factor-alpha (TNF-α) blockers, calcitonin gene related peptide antagonists, antimicrobials particularly in infectious cervical discitis and the traditional medicines including natural plants and herbs.

---

* E mail: alnimermarwan@ymail.com

I. INTRODUCTION

Cervical spine controls the head movement, therefore, a person's ability to direct his or her organs of sensation. When bone, muscles, or nerves of the neck region are damaged, activities ranged from sedentary to record-setting are disrupted. Approximately 10% of adults have neck pain at any one time. Neck pain is a highly prevalent condition among the general population. Data from cross-sectional studies show that point estimates range from 10% to 35% [Makela et al., 1991; Andersson et al., 1993; Côté et al., 1998]. The incidence rates increase with age up to 40 to 60 years, and then decrease slightly [Fejer et al., 2006; Bot et al., 2004]. Neck pain is generally more common in women than in men [Fejer et al., 2006; Bot et al., 2005]. Approximately 30% of people with neck pain face restrictions in their activities of daily living [Picavet and Schouten, 2003]. The prevalence of neck pain and disability is increased in individuals with a life time history of neck injury who are involved in a motor vehicle collision [Côté et al., 2000]. There are several possible causes of neck pain, although it is often difficult to know with certainty what is causing pain (Box 1).

Box 1. Causes of neck pain

Cervical strain
Cervical spondylosis
Cervical discogenic pain
Cervical facet syndrome
Whiplash injury
Cervical myofascial pain
Diffuse skeletal hyperostosis
Cervical spondylotic myelopathy
Cervical radiculopathy
Cervical herniated disc
Cervical osteoarthritis
Cervicogenic headache
Infection or osteomyelitis
Inflammatory rheumatologic disease
Vascular abnormality of cervical structures
Tumor or malignancy of cervical spine
Referred pain from cardiothoracic surgery
Psychogenic pain disorders
Malingering

This is because the examination, and even imaging tests, are not able easily differentiating among the various causes. It is often not necessary to determine the cause of a person's neck pain, especially if the pain is mild. In most cases, neck pain can be treated conservatively with Over-The-Counter (OCT) pain medications, ice, heat and massage and stretching exercise at home. Co-morbidities are frequently associated with disabling neck pain including headache, low back pain, cardiovascular events and gastrointestinal problems. The incidence of widespread pain disorders increases after cervical spinal injury. In a study of 161 cases of traumatic injury, fibromyalgia syndrome was 13 times more frequent after neck injury than after lower extremity injury [Buskila et al., 1997].

II. PAIN PERCEPTION

The definition of pain recommended by the International Association for the Study of Pain is that; it is an unpleasant sensory and emotional experience associated with actual or potential tissue damage [Merskey and Watson, 1979]. Allodynia is referred to pain in response to normally innocuous stimuli and if the intensity pain response is heightened, then it called hyperalgesia. Notiception is the detection of tissue damage by specialized receptors of Aδ and C nerve fibers. Acetylsalicylic acid and nonsteroidal anti-inflammatory drugs produce pain relief mainly by the restoration of nociceptive sensitivity to its resting state local and regional anaesthesia can prevent nociception from becoming pain. Pain due to nerve injury does not respond to analgesics such as morphine as efficiently as pain caused by tissue damage, indicating the complex relation between injury and pain.

Acute *vs* Chronic Pain

Acute neck pain is abrupt, intense pain that subsides after a period of days or weeks. It can also radiate to the head, shoulder, arms or hands. It typically resolves with rest, exercise, and other self-care measures. When it occurs, it is initially associated with specific autonomic and somatic reflexes, but these disappear in patients with chronic pain. It often relates to soft tissue injury (sprains of muscles, tendons, ligaments) or occurs suddenly and usually heals with several days or weeks. Its severity related directly to the extent of tissue injury and resolves overtime. Most people with acute neck pain respond rapidly to treatment and 90% are symptom free within 1-2 weeks. Recurrences of neck pain are common.

Chronic pain, such as low back pain, post herpetic neuralgia, fibromyalgia, are commonly triggered by an injury or disease, but may precipitated by factors other than the cause of pain. It is not the duration of pain that distinguish acute from chronic pain but, more importantly, the inability of the body to restore its physiological functions to normal homeostatic level. The intensity of the pain is out of proportion to the original injury or tissue damage. The intensity frequently bears little or no relation to the extent of tissue injury of other quantifiable pathology. All types of chronic pain lead people to seek health care but they are often not treated effectively. Chronic neck pain persists (lasts more than three months) and its source may be hard to determine. It continues despite treatment and inappropriate treatment of chronic pain runs as high as 50% [Sherman et al., 2006]. Chronic pain is common and represents a significant proportion of office visit complaints. Approximately 35% of the American population suffers from chronic pain and that is on the rise population ages [Sherman et al., 2006].

According to the nature of pain, it could be:

1. Nociceptive (inflammatory) pain. It is either somatic or visceral resulted from the consequence of trauma to peripheral tissue e.g. surgical incision, burn etc.

Nociceptive neurons become hyperexcitable leading to central sensitization and thus greater perception of pain in the higher centers. It may involve the abnormal pain state of allodynia or hyperalgesia that resulted from both peripheral and central hypersensitivity.

2. Neuropathic pain. It resulted from primary lesion or dysfunction in the nervous tissue e.g. nerve trans-section. It characterized by spontaneous pain, hyperalgesia and allodynia which can persist after the initial injury is resolved [Woolf and Mannion, 1999].
3. Psychogenic pain

According to the localization, the pain could be:

1. Localized neck pain generally points to muscle strains, ligament sprains and degenerative facet or disc processes.
2. Radiated neck pain that radiates into the upper limbs frequently stems from nerve involvement.

Mediators of Pain Perception

Some chemical mediators are produced at spinal level or released locally following tissue injury or inflammation. These mediators are involved in the perception of pain via direct activation of sensory nerve endings (e.g. proton, ATP, glutamate, 5-hydroxytryptamine, histamine and bradykinin) or indirectly through sensitization of the nerve ending to the action of other stimuli (e.g. prostaglandins and cytokines such as IL-1β, IL-2, IL-6, IL-8, TNF-α.). Sometimes these mediators express regulatory effect on the sensory neurons, adjacent inflammatory cells and sympathetic nerves e.g. bradykinin, tachykinins and nerve growth factors.

Central Mediators
The dorsal horn of the spinal cord contains many transmitters and receptors that involve in the spinal mechanism of perception. Examples of these transmitters are peptides (substance P, calcitonin gene related peptide (CGRP), somatostatin, neuropeptide Y, and galanin), inhibitory amino acids (gamma aminobutyric acid (GABA), glycine), excitatory amino acids (glutamate, aspartate), nitric oxide, arachidonic acid metabolites, adenosine, endogenous opioids, endogenous cannibinoids).

Peripheral Mediators
When the nociceptors in peripheral tissues are stimulated, the nociception pulses are transmitted to the central nervous system by two types of neurons; Aδ nerve fiber which transmit "first pain", sharp, prickling and injurious, and C- nerve fibers which responsible for "second pain" dull, aching and visceral. Various chemicals (bradykinin, histamine, serotonin, prostaglandins, potassium, proton) are released into damaged tissue cells of vascular origins (platelets, neutrophils, lymphocytes and macrophages) and also by mast cells. Some of these chemicals induce nociceptive reactions and can modify the activity of nociceptors either by

direct activation or by sensitization to different stimuli. Several mediators are involved in this mechanism. They include bradykinin, substances P, cytokines (interleukins, interferon, tumor necrosis factor) nerve growth factor, Prostaglandins, leukotriens, galanin, vasoactive intestinal peptide, somatostatin, cholecytokinin, Monoamines etc.

Neuropeptides

Neuropeptides include substance P, calitonin gene-related peptide, vasoactive intestinal peptide, nociceptin/orphanin FQ (N/OFQ). Local axon reflexes are responsible for the peripheral release of neuropeptides from sensory neurons leading to neurogenic inflammation [Suzuki et al., 1989]. Primary afferent fibers contained peptides which their profile is altered by sustained stimuli or damage to the nerve [Levine et al., 1993; Hökfelt et al, 1994]. In the spinal horn the peripheral noxious stimulation causes a release not only a substances P but also of other peptides such as neurokinin A (NKA), neurokonin B (NKB), calcitonin gene related peptide (CGRP) and somatostatin but not of galanin [Morton et al., 1988; Morton and Hutchison, 1989].

Substance P
It is synthesized in the spinal ganglion, from where it is transported centrally to the substantia gelatinosa of spinal dorsal horn and peripherally to the nerve endings in many tissues. Substance P occurs in small and medium sized neurons of substantia gelatinosa of the spinal dorsal horns, as well as in peripheral and central endings of primary afferent fibers. It is released by primary afferent nociceptive fibers at the level of spinal cord. It is believed that substance P together with other tachykinins is responsible for nociceptive transmission from the peripheral to the central nervous system [Iversen, 1982]. Intrathecal injection of substance P in mice elicits the behavior suggesting the pain sensation [Hylden and Wilcox, 1981], whereas tachykinin antagonists [Lembeck et al., 1981; Zubrzycka et al., 1997] administered by the same route produce an analgesic effect. Treatment with capsaicin resulted in a decrease in the substance P content in the dorsal horn and concomitant elevation of pain threshold [Nagy and Van Der Kooy, 1983]. The release of substance P is blocked by morphine at trigeminal level [Jessell and Iversen, 1977]. Blocking neurokinin-1 receptor does not alleviate the nociceptive effect of substance P [Mantyh et al., 1995; Mantyh et al., 1997]. Moreover, destruction of the neurons that express neurokinin-1 receptor led to a substantial reduction in allodynia and hyperalgesia induced by inflammation and nerve injury. Substance P appears to have a role in potentiating both excitatory and inhibitory inputs to spinal nociceptive neurons, an effect sensitizing the neurons to any synaptic input [Radhakrishnan and Henry, 1995].

Clinically substance P antagonists failed to relieve the pain in migraine and rheumatoid arthritis [Dray and Rang, 1998]. Substance P plays a role in neurogenic inflammation. It causes a degranulation of mast cells and thus the release of histamine, vasodilatation, and plasma extravasation with the subsequent release of other alogens (serotonin, bradykinin) and the activation of other inflammatory cells (macrophages, lymphocytes). Substance P also is able to induce production of nitric oxide from endothelium. Neurogenic inflammation also involves the release of substance P from sensory nerve endings in response to pain or infection. When the irritant capsaicin was applied to skin, edema occurred as a result of sensory neuropeptide release, including substance P [Iversen, 1998] Local administration of substance P had no effect on neuronal firing properties [Heppelmann and Pawlak, 1997]. Intense peripheral stimulation may induce release of substance P into the dorsal horn, causing central hyperexcitability and an increased sensitivity to pain [De Felipe et al., 1998]. Substance P and enkephalins exert opposite effects on the nociceptive neurons. Both somatostatin and galanin inhibit the release of substance P [Yangisawa et al., 1986].

Calcitonin Gene Related Peptide (CGRP)

It is derived, with calcitonin, from the CT/CGRP gene located on chromosome 11. It is a 37 amino acid peptide and is the most potent endogenous vasodilator currently known. CGRP was discovered when alternative processing of RNA transcripts from the calcitonin gene was shown to result in the production of distinct mRNAs encoding CGRP [Amara *et al.*, 1982]. It is primarily produced in nervous tissue however its receptors are expressed throughout the body. It is also strongly implicated in the vasodilatory effect of endogenous cannabinoid anandamide in the brain. CGRP enhances the release of substance P from primary afferent neuron [Oku et al., 1987]. CGRP has been shown to be important in the trigeminovascular system that is known to play an important role in the pathogenesis of migraine headache [Edvinsson, 2003; Olesen *et al.*, 2004]. This effect was found to be antagonised by capsazepine [Zygmunt et al., 1999]. In behavioural studies, CGRP has been shown to inhibit the antinociceptive effects produced by opioids [Welch *et al.*, 1989]. Since opioids produce analgesia, in part, by inhibiting the release of sensory transmitters in the spinal cord [Pohl *et al.*, 1989], an adaptative increase in the release of a neuropeptides such as CGRP could physiologically antagonize opioid action and thus lead to the development of tolerance. The combination of a CGRP receptor antagonist with morphine presents an option for the inhibition of clinical tolerance and may provide a new avenue for restoring opioid responsiveness in neuropathic pain states. Hyperresponsivness of sensory neurons following acute synovitis could be blocked by the selective antagonist $CGRP_{8-37}$ [Neugebauer et al., 1996]. Local application of capsaicin onto the sciatic nerve can alleviate mechanical hyperalgesia in a peripheral neuropathic pain models as a result of decrease of TRPV1- and CGRP-positive sensory [Kim et al., 2008]. In the spinal cord, proteasome inhibitors abolished the enhanced capsaicin-evoked calcitonin gene-related peptide (CGRP) release and dynorphin A upregulation, both elicited by nerve injury suggesting the involvement of CGRP in chronic pain [Ossipov et al., 2007].

Tachykinins

Tachykinin peptides are neuropeptides, found from amphibians to mammals. They were so named due to their ability to rapidly induce contraction of gut tissue [Carter and Krause, 1990]. The two human tachykinin genes are called TAC1 and TAC3 for historical reasons, and are equivalent to Tac1 and Tac2 of the mouse, respectively.

The broad term tachykinin refers to a family of neuropeptides that have a common C-terminal amino acid sequence with a varying N-terminal sequence and substance P-like activity. Of the many tachykinins found in nature, only those found in mammals are referred to as neurokinins. In addition to substance P there are other two neurokinins; neurokinin A (NKA) and neurokinin B (NKB) [Vaught, 1988]. Neurokinin A (NKA), formerly known as substance K, is a member of the tachykinin family of neuropeptide neurotransmitters. It is produced from the same preprotachykinin gene as the neuropeptide substance P. The release of NKA by noxious stimuli in the dorsal horn is more widely spread and longer lasting than that of substance P [Duggan et al., 1990].

Neurokinin 1 (NK1) receptors have the greatest affinity for substance P. Substance P is considered to be the primary nociceptive transmitter in afferent sensory fibers, released in response to noxious cutaneous stimuli and participating in conduction across sensory afferent nerves (C-fibers). Selective destruction of neurokinin-1 receptor in the superfacial spinal cord leads to a sustained reduction in allodynia and hyperalgesia induced by inflammation and nerve injury.

Tachykinins include: neurokinin A, neurokinin K, neuropeptide gamma and substance P [Dornan et al., 1993]. There are three known mammalian tachykinin receptors termed NK1, NK2 and NK3. The receptors are not specific to any individual tachykinin, they do have differing affinity for the tachykinins:

NK1: Substance P>Neurokinin A>Neurokinin B

NK2: Neurokinin A > Neurokinin B > Substance P

NK3: Neurokinin B > Neurokinin A > Substance P

Galanin

It is a neuropeptide present in humans and other mammals. It involved in a number of physiological processes including nociception, response to nerve injury and peripheral inflammation [Liu and Hökfelt, 2002]. It is predominantly an inhibitory, hyperpolarizing neuropeptide and as such inhibits neurotransmitter release. It is often co-localized with substance P and calcitonin gene related peptide. Galanin is expressed in dorsal root ganglion at relatively low levels in <5% of small-diameter C fiber type [Hökfelt et al., 1987]. It might play a role in the regulation of inflammation and nociception. The role of galanin in pain signaling is complex. In intact nerves, exogenously applied galanin have both facilitatory and inhibitory effects on nociception [Kuraishi et al., 1991; Post et al., 1988]. Galanin is a strongly inhibitory, hyperpolarizing peptide, which reduces the excitability of its target cells. Galanin, acting at the three galanin receptors, opens ATP-sensitive potassium channels, closes calcium channels (N- and L-types), modifies intracellular calcium levels, reduces the stimulatory effect of muscarinic agonists on phospholipase C and modulates the activity of adenylyl cyclase. Activation of galanin receptor-1 inhibits the release of substance P and alleviates allodynia. Several studies have shown that intrathecal galanin significantly reduces allodynia induced by chronic constriction injury [Liu and Hökfelt, 2000; Yu et al., 1999]. In addition, Eaton et al. [1999] have shown that a spinal cord implant of genetically modified cells that secrete galanin significantly reduces allodynia after chronic constriction injury. It has been found that the concentration of galanin was significantly lower in the ankles and spinal cords of rats with adjuvant arthritis compared to controls [Qinyang et al., 2004].

Vasoactive Intestinal Peptide (VIP)

It is a 28 amino acid neuropeptide that is contained in postganglionic sympathetic as well as capsaicin–sensitive sensory nerve fibers [Ahmed et al., 1995]. VIP6-28 (VIP antagonist) reduced nociceptive and pain levels in rat model of osteoarthritis [McDougall and Watkins, 2006].

Somatosstatin

It is found in cells of dorsal root ganglion and in afferent terminals of the dorsal horn. It released in response to noxious stimuli leading to hyperpolarization and reduced firing rate in dorsal horn cells. Intrathecal administration of somatostatin produces analgesia and motor dysfunction [Mollenholt, 1988].

Endogenous Opioids

Numerous regions of the brain are rich in opioid peptides and the mRNAs for the opioid receptors [Mansour et al., 1996]. The supraspinal actions of opioids have a key role in the analgesic effects of systemic morphine. Moreover, opioids shared in peripheral antinociception in hyperalgesic inflammatory conditions [Stein and Yassouridis, 1997]

Endogenous Cannobinoids

The endocannobinoid anandamide is enzymatically synthesized from free arachidonic acid and ethanolamine [Deutsch and Chin, 1993]. Anandamide is a nonselective ligand that binds to both CB1 and CB2 cannobinoid G-protein-coupled receptors. The activation of these receptors could modulate pain generation and perception [Pertwee, 2001]. Anandamide activates the transient receptor potential vanilloid channel 1 (TRPV1), causing secondary release of CGRP [Zygmunt et al., 1999].

Nociceptin/Orphanin FQ (N/OFQ)

It is an opioid like neuropeptide that has been immunolocalized in the peripheral and central neurons systems where it controls central pain mechanism [Civelli et al., 1998; Darland et al., 1998]. It is able to induce hyperalgesia and allodynia in the joint [McDougall et al., 2006] as a result of secondary release of substance P into the joint. Selective NK1-receptor antagonist RP67580 blocked N/OFQ mediated nociception [McDougall et al., 2001].

Glutamate

It released by primary afferent fibers and had an important role in the spinal mechanisms of pain transmission. Various receptors and subtypes are involved at the spinal level (AMPA, metabotrophic, kainite). The NMDA receptor is important in the synaptic events that lead to central sensitivity and hyperalgesia [Dickenson, 1995; Urban et al., 1994].The release of substance P into the spinal cord on afferent stimulation removes the magnesium block of the channel of the NMDA-receptor in range of persistent pain state. Activation of NMDA receptors leads to an entry of calcium into the neuron which can then produce other mediators from spinal nerves by increasing the activity of enzymes e.g. nitric oxide synthase, phospholipase A2 [Malmberg and Yaksh, 1992a]

Inhibitory Amino Acids

Glycine and γ-aminobutyric acid (GABA) act at dorsal horn controlling the NMDA receptors and they might play a role in etiology of neuropathic pain. Blockade of spinal GABA or glycine can result in allodynia [Yaksh, 1989]. Up-regulation of spinal GABA receptors occurred when there is peripheral inflammation, to promote inhibition of afferent nociceptive impulses and decrease pain sensation [Dickenson, 1995].

Monoamines

Nociceptive impulses activating the sympathetic nervous system promote norepinephrine releases which in turn accelerates sensitization of the nociceptors creating another vicious cycle [Dray, 1995]. Serotonin is a major inflammatory mediator, especially in the initial phase of inflammatory process [Capasso et al., 1975]. It causes direct activation of sensory neurons via 5HT3 receptor activation. As a result of activation of 5HT2 and 5HT3 receptors, the peripheral nociceptors are activated and producing hyperalgesia and neurogenic inflammation [Richardson et al., 1985; Barnes et al., 1990; Rueff and Dray, 1993]. On the other hand, activation of $5HT_{1B}$ and $5HT_{1D}$ receptors decreases pain and inflammation. In the periphery $5HT_{1B}$ and $5HT_{1D}$ agonists inhibit neurogenic inflammation [Zochodne and Ho, 1994].

Free Radical

Reactive oxygen species such as hydrogen peroxide, hydroxyl radical are produced by tissue during inflammation. They enhance the effects of bradykinin, prostaglandin E2 and other inflammatory mediators. Nitric oxide has been implicated in the degeneration of intervertebral disc. Elevated nitric oxide production has been found in cerebrospinal fluid in patients with degenerative lumbar disease [Podichetty, 2007]. The level of nitric oxide was significantly higher in the herniated cervical disc specimens obtained from patients undergoing discectomy for persistent radiculopathy compared with the control discs [Kang et al., 1995]. In cervicogenic headache, a unilateral headache that provoked by neck movement or pressure on tender points in the neck, the nitrogen species radicals were significantly elevated in serum during the periods of headache [Inan et al., 2007]. Nitric oxide in a complex way exacerbates the noxious transmission. Intracutaneous injection of nitric oxide provoke pain in human [Holthuusen and Arndt, 1994]. On the other hand topical nitric oxide donor in form of transdermal glyceryl trinitrate preparation improved the clinical outcome of patient with chronic extensor tendinosis at the elbow [Paoloni et al., 2003].

Purines

The receptors for the purines, notably the P2X3 (a ligand-gated ion channel triggered by ATP) which is selectively expressed by small diameter sensory neurons. ATP infusion into trapezius muscle induces strong pain and local tenderness in healthy man. ATP induces sustained facilitation of craniofacial nociception by prolonged excitation of P2X3 receptors in neck muscles [Makowska et al., 2006]. Sole administration 100 nmol/L ATP facilitates brainstem nociception in mice and it reversed by local application of tetradotoxin in neck muscles [Ellrich and Makowska, 2007].

Bradykinin

It is a powerful alogenic substance released from kininogen in a way that is dependent on protein kinase C and calcium and sensitizes nociceptors by means of activation of postganglionic sympathetic neurons which then produce PGE2. Bradykinin involved in release of prostaglandins, cytokines, free radicals, histamine from degranualted mast cell and stimulation of sympathetic neurons leading to vasodilatation.

Histamine

It is released from mast cells during degranulation, a process promoted by substance P, kinins, interleukin-1, and nerve growth factor. It acts on sensory neurons to produce pain and itching [Simone et al, 1991]. Histamine stimulation of sensory neurons may evoke release neuropeptides and prostaglandins.

Cytokines (Interleukins, Interferon, And Tumor Necrosis Factor)

They are released by phagocytes and cells of the immune system, and have an important role in the inflammatory process. Bradykinin plays a role in the production of cytokines [Dray, 1997]. Some of these cytokines are powerful inflammatory mediators that can activate sensory neuron through different mechanisms, some of which include sympathetic nervous system.

Nerve Growth Factor (NGF)

Central actions, mediated by changes in the expression of neuropeptides, ion channels, and growth factors in the sensory neurons, contribute to later manifestations [Donnerer et al., 1992; Leslie et al., 1995; Michael et al., 1997]. It is upregulated by inflammatory process. It has a key role in the development of sensory and autonomic neuron and process of nociception. It is produced by fibroblast and schwan cells and then increases the excitability of nociceptors which lead to hyperalgesia.

Eicosanoids

Eicosanoids are lipid membrane derived metabolites of arachidonic acid that include prostaglandins, leucotriens, lipoxins, thromboxanes and endocannobinoids. The pain field has generally focused on the activity of cyclooxygenases (COX) of which there are two isoforms COX-1 and COX-2. COX-1 enzyme is constitutively expressed in most cells where its function to maintain normal physiological process in tissues. COX-2 enzyme is present at the site of inflammation (i.e. inducible). Prostaglandins are weak alogens (pain producing) but play major part in the sensitization of receptors to other substances reducing their activation threshold [Birrell et al., 1991; Cohen and Perl, 1990]. Prostaglandin E2 stimulates neurons directly, initiating the transmission of pain impulses along nociceptive pathways. COX -2 enzyme can be produced by different signals mediating cytokines. The antiiinflammatory and antinoceptive effects of COX-2 inhibitors seems to be equivalent to those of non selective COX-2 inhibitors, but the main advantage of COX-2 inhibition will be the absence of gastric side effects in patients with chronic pain of inflammatory origin.

Lipoxins

Lipoxins were first described by Serhan, Hamberg and Samuelsson in 1984. Lipoxins are derived enzymatically from arachidonic acid. Lipoxin, signaling through the lipoxin A4 receptor, inhibits chemotaxis, transmigration, superoxide generation and NF-κB activation (Chiang et al., 2005). Lipoxins are high affinity antagonists to the cysteinyl leukotriene receptor type 1 (CysLT1) to which several leukotrienes (LTC_4, LTD_4 and LTE_4) mediate their smooth muscle contraction and eosinophil chemotactic effects.

Various chemical mediators are involved in turning off inflammation and pain. Lipoxins are one such class mediators that have been formed to act as "braking signals" in inflammation. Lipoxins reduce inflammation when administered directly to the inflamed area or given systematically (intravenously or orally). Acetylsalicylic acid triggers the release of lipoxins as one of its mechanism in reducing inflammation. Lipoxins have central and peripheral effects. Svensson et al [2007] showed that intravenous or intraspinal lipoxins injections can alter pain processing and reduce the pain sensitivity in rats. Local anti-inflammatory effect is observed with intravenous lipoxins injection.

Lipoxin A_4 and aspirin-triggered lipoxin A_4 are anti- inflammatory, proresolving possess, and modulate leukotrienes, cytokines, and chemokines [Serhan, 2005]. LXA_4 and its receptor are present in human osteoarthritis and synovitis of rheumatoid arthritis [Marcouiller et al., 2005; Hashimoto et al., 2007]. Human synovial fibroblasts express ALX, and, at nanomolar concentrations, LXA_4 reduces the levels of inflammatory cytokines and matrix metalloproteinases in synovial fibroblasts stimulated with interleukin 1β, as well as stimulating tissue inhibitors of metalloproteinase- 1[Sodin-Semrl, 2000;2004].

Resolvins and Protectins

These compounds are made by the human body from the omega-3 fatty acids eicosapentaenoic acid and docosahexaenoic acid. They are produced by the COX-2 pathway especially in the presence of aspirin. These mediators have anti-inflammatory and pro-resolution properties, thereby protecting organs from collateral damage, stimulating the clearance of inflammatory debris and promoting mucosal antimicrobial defense [Serhan et al., 2008]. Experimental evidence indicates that resolvins reduce cellular inflammation by inhibiting the production and transportation of inflammatory cells and chemicals to the sites of inflammation. Resolvin E1, at very low amounts reduces polymorph nuclear cells migration, dermal inflammation and interleukin-12 production [Serhan et al., 2002; Arita et al., 2005]. Resolvins and protectins transforming growth factor-β and growth factors produced by macrophages, also have a crucial role in the resolution of inflammation, including the initiation of tissue repair [Serhan and Savill, 2005; Serhan, 2007].

Ions Channel Ligands

Multiple different types of ion channels exist on the terminals of nociceptors. They are activated either directly or via coupling process. These channels:

a. *Acid sensing ion channel.* Acid sensing ion channel closely match the proton-gated cation channel described in sensory neurons. It is expressed in dorsal root ganglia and is also distributed widely throughout the brain. It is rapidly activated by condition of acidity below pH 6.5 [Waldmann et al., 1997].
b. *Sodium channel.* Up-regulation of sodium channels expression is observed in chronic inflammation [Black et al., 2004]. Inflammatory mediators (PGs, adenosine, 5HT) augment the sodium channel kinetics and tetrodotoxin-resistant current [England et al., 1996].These mediators facilitate transmission of action potentials by modification of the voltage threshold of several ion channels including the tetrodotoxin–resistant sodium channels. Therefore sodium channel blockers like mexilitine and crobenetine inhibit mechanical hyperalgesia [Laird et al., 2001].
c. *TRP channel.* Of particular interest in pain research are TRPM (melanostatin) and the TRMV (vanilloid) channels subfamilies. The eight member of the TRPM channel (TRPM8) is activated by cooling temperature (22-26°C). Pharmacological activation

of TRPM8 channel could elicit an antinociceptive effect. The ion channel responsible for noxious thermo-sensation is TRPV1 [Caterina et al., 1997]. TRPV1-channel is activated by temperature above 43°C, proton, lipids, phorbols and cannobinoids. Capsaicin sensitizes afferent neurons by secondary release of inflammation peptides.

III. CENTRAL, TOPICAL AND PERIPHERALLY ACTING ANALGESICS

Several drug categories are included in the management of neck pain. Their effects are either centrally or peripherally or sometimes at both levels. The majority of these drugs are prescribed to alleviate pain and muscle spasm or to stabilize the nerve function. In certain occasion, drugs combination is prescribed for the purpose of synergism and in other situation intrathecal injection is necessary to combat the neck pain. The following drug categories are currently used in the management of neck pain:

A. Nonsteroidal Anti-Inflammatory Drugs (NSAIDs)

The prostaglandins are implicated in various physiological and pathophysiological events. The prostanoid family includes PGD2, PGE2, PGF2α, Thromboxane A2 and prostaglandins. The biosynthesis of prostaglandins and some other prostanoids is catalyzed in a rate limiting step by PG-H synthase (COX), PG-endoperoxidase synthase which converts arachidonic acid to prostaglandin/prostanoid precursor PGH2. More than three cyclogenases isoenzymes are characterized. These are:

COX-1 (human 576aa, 69-72kDa; chromosome 9), COX-2 (human, 604aa, 74 kDa ; chromosome 1), COX-3 (canine 633aa, 65kDa in human aorta), COX-1 derived-proteins or partial COX-1 (PCOX1a; canine 414aa, 53kDa in human aorta and PCOX1b).

COX-1, a constitutively expressed isoform, produces physiologically relevant prostanoids such as in stomach and platelets. COX-2 is inducible and rapidly up-regulated at inflammation sites and forms proinflammatory prostanoids (Box 2). Prostanoids sensitize peripheral nociceptor terminals and produce localized pain hypersensitivity

In 1971, professor John Vane from Cornell University was awarded the Nobel Prize for his work in elucidating the mechanism of action of aspirin on prostaglandins [cited from Marienfeld et al., 1997]. Nonsteroidal anitiinflammatory drugs reduce the formation of prostaglandins by inhibiting the activity of COX-1, COX-2 and COX-3.

Box 2. Expression of COX isoform enzymes

Arachidonic acid		
COX-1	COX-2	COX-3
Prostaglandins production		
Gastric protection Platelet activation	Inducible inflammation	Pain and fever

Possible effects (mechanisms) for the analgesic activity of NSAID include:

1. Peripheral actions via:

- Altering stimulation of sensory nerve endings. NSAIDs reduce prostaglandins production leading to block the nociception response to endogenous mediators of inflammation, with the effect being greater in tissues that have been subjected to injury and trauma [Kitahata, 1993]. Also they inhibit prostaglandin-mediated sensitization of nociceptors to chemical and mechanical irritants [Dahl and Kehlet, 1991].
- Interfering with membrane signal transduction. They stabilize the cell membrane, an effect may account for the decrease in prostaglandins release.
- Interfering with bradykinin activity.

2. Central actions via:

- Interfering with prostaglandins synthesis
- Altering transmission of impulses by nerves that release substance P or CGRP
- Causing the release of endogenous opioid (enkephalin) or GABA, leading to impulse transmission block.
- Intrathecal adminstration of NSAIDs have been shown to reduce hyperalgesia [Malmberg and Yaksh, 1992b]. NSAIDs affect the synthesis of substances thought to play role in the processing of nociceptive impulses in the dorsal horn like serotonin, kynuremic acid and polyamines [McCormack, 1994].

3. Other possible mechanisms of action of NSAIDs in inhibiting inflammation

1. Alter neutrophil function
2. Interfere with mitochondrial function, alters oxidative phosphorylation, decrease ATP.
3. Stabilize lysosomal membranes.
4. Interfere with kinin formation and/or activity
5. Inhibit the activity of selecins.
6. Inhibit $NF-k_B$ formation ($NF-k_B$ is important in production and stimulation of cytokines)

Classification of COX inhibitors (Tables 1 and 2)

1. Selective COX-1: COX-1 inhibitor with not measurable effects of COX-2 activity e.g. low doses of acetylsalicylic acid (potent inhibitor at concentration 0.1 mM). Sodium salicylate is very weak inhibitor of COX-1.
2. Nonselective COX: Minimal differences between dose-response curves inhibition of either COX-1 or COX-2.
3. Preferential COX-2: It appears to produce its pharmacological effects on COX-2 at doses that have minimal effects on COX-1. However, high doses inhibit COX-1.
4. Selective COX-2: It only inhibits COX-2 at maximum therapeutic dose. Increasing dose should not result in significant inhibition of COX-1.

Table 1. IC$_{50}$ values for the inhibition of COX-1 and COX-2 in human whole blood assay

Drug	IC$_{50}$ (COX-1) µM	IC$_{50}$ (COX-2) µM	COX-1/COX-2 ratio
Indomethacin	0.19	0.44	0.4
Ibuprofen	4.8	24.3	0.2
6-MNA metabolite	28.9	154	0.2
Piroxicam	0.76	9.0	0.2
Etodolac	9.0	3.7	2.4
Meloxicam	1.4	7.0	2.0
Diclofenac	0.15	0.05	3.0
Celecoxib	6.7	0.87	7.7
Valdecoxib	26.1	0.87	30
Etoricoxib	116	1.1	106

Table 2. IC$_{50}$ values for the inhibition of COX-1 and COX-2 in intact cells

Drug	IC$_{50}$ (COX-1) µM	IC$_{50}$ (COX-2) µM	COX-1/COX-2 ratio
Acetylsalicylic acid	1.67	278	166
Sulindac	1.12	112	100
Indomethacin	0.03	1.68	60
Sodium salicylate	254	725	2.8
Acetaminophen	17.9	133	2.4
Valdecoxib	26.1	0.87	0.03

The following general notes should be taken in consideration when NSAIDs are prescribed vto patients with neck pain:

1. They reduce pain at low doses and decrease inflammation at high doses.
2. Once-a-day dosing is preferable to improve compliance.
3. Salicylic acid in pharmaceutical preparation of aspirin is rarely indicated because an irreversible inhibition of cyclogeneases.
4. All NSAIDs have a dose-related ceiling point for analgesia.
5. The efficacy of COX-2 inhibitors is the same with the noselective inhibitors.

NSAIDs in lower dosages and a less regular schedule is more likely to utilize the analgesic properties. In single dose, most of NSAIDs are effective analgesics than a single dose of acetaminophen or acetylsalicylic acid. The analgesic actions of NSAIDs can be dissociated from the anti-inflammatory effect, and this may reflect additional spinal and supraspinal actions of NSAIDs to inhibit various aspect of central pain processing [Yaksh et al., 1998]. Both COX- isoforms (COX-1 and COX-2) contribute to spinal and supraspinal prostanoid production following tissue injury or inflammation [Yaksh et al., 1998]. Moreover, NSAIDs had effect upon the healing of the injured soft tissue, namely muscle and tendon. In vitro model of isolated human fibroblast subjected to repeated motion injury, indomethacin accelerates the protein synthesis during the later remodeling phase of healing [Almekinders et al., 1995].

Celecoxib, COX-2 inhibitor, showed better scores than sustained release acetaminophen for pain, stiffness and functional limitation in patients with osteoarthritis in multiple sites [Yelland et al., 2006]. COX-2 inhibitors have been associated with cardiovascular toxicity. Rofecoxib was withdrawn from the worldwide market because of this effect, demonstrated in the APPROVE trial. This trial was conducted at 108 centers worldwide with recruitment in 2000 and 2001, and examined the protective effect of rofecoxib on adenomatous polyps but was terminated early because of cardiovascular toxicity [Baron et al., 2008]. The use of 25 mg/day rofecoxib is associated with increased risk for cardiovascular event which persists to one year after treatment is stopped.

Topical NSAIDs

When NSAIDs are administered topically, relatively high concentrations occur in the dermis, where levels in the muscle are at least equivalent to those following systemic administration [Heyneman et al., 2000]. Topically applied NSAIDs do reach the synovial fluid, but it is not clear whether this effect reflect local penetration or results from systemic circulation [Vaile and Davis, 1998]. In human topical application of NSAIDs produces analgesia in models of cutaneous pain [McCormack et al., 2000] and muscle pain [Steen et al., 2000]. The effect of topical NSAIDs in osteoarthritis and rheumatoid arthritis varied between 18-92% [Heyneman et al., 2000].

Topical application of NSAIDs may be useful for acute inflammation and localized pain. In experimental animal model patch sheets of loxoprofen sodium, felbinac, indomethacin or ketoprofen have analgesic effects, inhibit expression of c-Fos in the dorsal horn (loxoprofen sodium and indomethacin), and reduce PGE2 levels (loxoprofen sodium in inflamed tissues [Sekiguchi et al., 2008]. Adverse reactions of topical NSAIDs are cutaneous which occur in 10-15% of patient in form of skin rash and pruritis at the site of application [Moore et al., 1998] and less likely systemic adverse reactions.

B. Acetaminophen: The Para-Amino Phenol Derivative

It is the active metabolite of phenacetin a so called coal tar analgesic. In vivo, phenacetin is converted to acetaminophen. In 1852 Gerhardt discovered acetaminophen that reducing fever and pain. It was first used in clinical medicine in 1893 but wide spread use began after its FDA approval in 1950. It is effective as an analgesic and antipyretic. It has a weak anti-inflammatory action; possibly due to its weak inhibition of cyclooxygenase (as measured in the presence of high concentrations of peroxides found in inflammatory lesions) and hence its weak inhibition of prostaglandin synthesis. Acetaminophen has a unique activity profile based in part on its action at its molecular targets, the cyclooxygenase enzyme that produces prostaglandins responsible for pain, fever and inflammation. COX-3 (a COX enzyme isoform encoded by COX-1 gene) is sensitive to selective inhibition by acetaminophen that reduces pain and fever but has weak anti-inflammatory (Chandrasekharan et al., 2002; Warner and Mitchel, 2002). Therefore, its efficacy as an analgesic may be less than other nonsteroidal anti-inflammatory drugs like aspirin. COX-3 is also the target for diclofenac, aspirin and ibuprofen.

In therapeutic doses, acetaminophen inhibits the activity of COX-3 enzyme while in toxic doses it activates nuclear receptor (CAR) leading to expression of three cytochrome P450 enzymes that transform acetaminophen into a reactive toxic metabolites, NAPOI which responsible for hepatotoxicity. Acetaminophen is primarily centrally acting, has no effect on platelet aggregation, and is reversible inhibitor of cyclooxygenase enzyme. In experimental animal model, pretreatment of rats with oral acetaminophen significantly attenuated intrathecal substance P-induced hyperalgesia and suppressed the release of spinal PGE2 [Crawley et al., 2008]. Also intrathecal acetaminophen produces dose dependent antinoceptive effect indicating the central hyperalgesic action of acetaminophen. The antipyretic activity is exerted by blocking the effect of endogenous pyrogens on the hypothalamic heat-regulation center possibly by inhibiting prostaglandins synthesis. Analgesic effect of acetaminophen may be produced by direct action on the pain threshold. This effect is believed to be due to inhibition of prostaglandins and/or inhibition of the synthesis or actions of chemical mediators or other substances that sensitize the pain receptors to mechanical or chemical stimulation.

It is the preferred analgesic for patients with osteoarthritis and other conditions associated with minor pain. One survey estimated that nearly 3% of all Americans over 20 years old are frequent monthly users of acetaminophen [Paulose-Ram et al., 2005].

Acetaminophen is being more effective than placebo in relieving pain of large joint osteoarthritis but NSAIDs and coxibs show superior efficacy to acetaminophen and are also effective for stiffness [Neame et al., 2004; Zhang et al., 2004; Pincus et al., 2004].

The hazard ratio for hospitalization for a gastrointestinal event was 1.2 for patients taking more than 3g /day acetaminophen; 1.63 for those taking NSAIDs and 2.55 for those taking combination of NSAIDs and more than 3g/day of acetaminophen [Rahme et al., 2008]. Acetaminophen is able to exert analgesic effect in nociceptive tests that are sensitive to central analgesics and in which there is no inflammation [Bustamante et al., 1996]. In the rat formalin test, significant reduction in the antinoceceptive action of acetaminophen is observed when the serotonergic bulbospinal pathways are damages or there is depletion in serotonin level [Pini et al., 1996]. Intrathecal administration of 5HT receptor antagonists inhibit the antinociceptive action of acetaminophen suggesting that the inhibition occurred as the spinal level by means of a serotonergic mechanism [Courade et al ., 2001]. Moreover, intrathecal injection of selective 5HTA1 receptor antagonist (WAY-100635) reversed the action of acetaminophen in the rat formalin test suggesting that its antinociceptive activity depends on the stimulation of the spinal $5HT_{A1}$ receptor [Bonnefont et al., 2003; 2005]. Bonnefont et al [2007] showed that specific $5-HT_{A1}$ receptor-dependent cellular events in acetaminophen produced antinociception, and the inhibition of COX activities is not the exclusive mechanism involved.

C. Opioids

Presynaptic opioid receptors decrease the release of excitatory neurotransmitters from nociceptive neurons, specifically the neurons that send small C-fibers and Aδ fibers into the periphery and respond to a variety of noxious stimuli. Postsynaptic pioid receptors have similar effects on the second-order neuron. Opioids exert their analgesic effects by binding to and activating receptors that comprise part of an endogenous opioid system. There are three distinct families of endogenous opioid peptides: the endorphins (interact with μ and δ receptors), the enkephalins (interact with δ receptors), and the dynorphins (interact with κ receptors). Also two additional short peptides that display a high affinity and selectivity for μ opioid receptors have been identified. These peptides; endomorphin-1 and endomorphin-2, produce potent and prolonged analgesia in animals. Most recently, a receptor that is structurally similar to the opioid receptor was discovered. This receptor has been classified as opioid-receptor-like 1 (ORL1). The natural ligand has been termed orphanin FQ (OFQ), or nociceptin. It appears to be involved in the central modulation of pain. Opioid receptors that are capable of mediating analgesia in humans have been discovered on peripheral sensory nerve terminals and are very similar to those of receptors in the brain. The prevailing peptides found in the periphery are the endorphins and enkephalins. This peripheral opioid system interacts with immune functions. In brief the supraspinal and peripheral analgesia produced by opioid are related to:

1. *mu*-and/or δ receptor agonists reduce release primary afferent neurotransmitters (substance P, glutamate) from C-fibers and inhibited the release of CGRP [Dickenson,1986; Kangrga and Randić, 1991].
2. *mu*-receptor agonists prevent the nociceptor sensitization by PGE2 by μ-receptor agonist [Levine and Taiwo, 1989]. Also delta and kappa receptor agonists block bradykinin-induced release of nocoiceptor sensitizing agents from the nerve ending [Taiwo and Levine, 1991]. Intraarticular injection of morphine before the procedure of arthroscopy appears to be more effective than after arthroscopy. This supports the importance of preemptive inhibition of peripheral inflammatory and hyperalgesia pathway [Denti, 1997]. Topical application of opioid to somatic site may also produces analgesia in number of experimental models [Nozaki-Taguchi and Yaksh, 1999].
3. Opioid will delay the onset of wind-up phenomenon.
4. Antiinflammatory property, opioid reduced the synovial leucocytes count, may have contributed to the pain relief [Martinez et al., 1996].

Opioids are very effective in reducing the severity of spine pain and in producing pain relief. Dosage escalations are typically related to an identifiable worsening of the painful condition, a surgical complication or an unrelated pain process [Mahowald et al., 2005].

Oxycodone (controlled release) therapy significantly improved the quality of life and quality of sleep in patients with refractory and frequent acute episodes of chronic neck pain who failed to respond to non-opioid conservative treatment [Ma et al., 2007]. Patients with chronic neck pain due to facet cervical joint pain were responded to fentanyl better than midazolam sedation [Manchikanti et al., 2004a]. Chao et al [2005] observed that oral morphine (sustained release) reduced the main pain score in patients with lower back pain with radiculoneuropathy, neck pain, headache, degenerative disc disease, failed back syndrome, and radiculoneuropathies and its use did not result in escalation of dose strength or frequency, and was safe and efficacious regardless of patient age. Small-dose ketamine improved the analgesic effects of fentanyl patient controlled analgesia after cervical surgery and to a less extent after lumbar surgery [Yamauchi et al., 2008]. The quality of emergence from anesthesia in patients with cervical spine surgery is improved with fentanyl-based anesthesia [Inoue et al., 2005].

Opioid therapy should be considered in severe cervical spondylosis as the preferred treatment since of addiction during therapy is less than 1%.

Long term opioid treatment for nonmalignant pain is not appropriate for the large majority of patients, and that most patients do worse, not better [Schofferman, 1993].

Transdermal Fentanyl

Use of transdermal fentanyl in chronic non malignant pain is controversial. Patients with low back pain can be successfully given transdermal fentanyl with similar or improved control pain [Jeal and Benfield, 1997]. Data from open, randomized, parallel group multicenter study included 680 patients with chronic low back pain showed that transdermal fentanyl and sustained release morphine provided similar levels of pain relief besides that transdermal fentanyl is associated with significantly less constipation than sustained release morphine [Allan et al., 2005]. Patients with neuropathic pain temporarily responded to intravenous fentanyl and good prolonged pain control with tolerable side effects [Dellemijn and Vanneste, 1997]. In a 16-week open-label study evaluated pre- and postdrug therapy effects, Agarwal et al [2007] found that significant reduction in pain intensity and increase in daytime activity in chronic neuropathic pain patients treated with transdermal fentanyl.

Opioid and Dependence

Neck pain was estimated in relation to analgesic consumption at baseline. Individuals who reported use of analgesics daily or weekly at baseline showed significant increased risk for having chronic pain and analgesic overuse at follow-up but it was less evident than individuals with chronic migraine [Zwart et al., 2003]. Persons with chronic spinal pain were at elevated risk to have chronic pain at other anatomic sites, to have a range of medical comorbidities, and to have mood and substance use disorders [Gureje et al., 2007].

Chronic pain and prolonged use of opioids raise the prevalence of opioids dependence in spine surgery patients to 20% [Walid et al., 2007]. In that study, thirty patients were opioid dependent among 150 spine surgery patients [48 lumbar diskectomy, 60 cervical decompression and fusion and 42 lumbar decompression and fusion]. And the prevalence was highest among lumbar decompression and fusion patients and among females, and was positively correlated with pain intensity. Opioid tolerance to the peripheral analgesia may developed [Aley et al., 1995], and it reversed or even prevented by NMDA receptor antagonists [Kolensnikov and Pasternak, 1999]. Studies of opioids for nonmalignant pain have shown minimal risk of addiction or abuse behaviors in patients with neuropathic pain [Watson and Babul, 1998].

On the other hand narcotic abuse is considered as a cause of neck pain. There is a high risk of cervical osteomyelitis in intravenous drug abusers due to the use of jugular veins for administration of drugs. Rapid vertebral body destruction at any cervical levels secondary to cervical osteomyelitis in an intravenous drug abuser was reported [Arun et al., 2007; Singh et al., 2006]. Advanced vertebral body destruction, disk space infection, prevertebral abscess, and anterior cervical inflammatory reaction appear to be typical findings on radiographs in heroin abusers with cervical osteomyelitis [Endress et al., 1990]. Schreiber and Formal [2007] reported spinal cord infarction in the anterior spinal artery distribution in woman recreationally inhaled cocaine presented with neck pain and muscle weakness.

D. Capsaicinoids and Vanilloids Agonists

Capsaicin
Dihydrocapsaicin
Nordihydrocapsaicin
Homodihydrocapsaicin
Homocapsaicin
Nonivamide

Capsaicin

Capsaicin is the active component of chili peppers which are plants belonging to the genus Capsicum. It produces burning sensation in any tissue with which comes in contact. Pure capsaicin is a hydrophobic, colorless, odorless, crystalline- waxy compound. It was first isolated in 1816 in crystalline form by P.A. Bucholz and again 30 years later by L.T. Thresh who give it the name capsaicin. It was first synthesized in 1930 by E. Spath and F.S. Darling. In 1961, similar substances were isolated from chili peppers by the Japanese chemists S. Kosuge and Y. Inagaki who named them capsaicinoids [Kosuge et al., 1961; Kosuge and Inagaki1962].

Capsaicin is currently used in topical ointments to relieve the pain of peripheral neuropathy (postherpetic neuralgia). It may be used as creams for the temporarily relief of minor aches and pains of muscles and joints associated with arthritis, simple backache, strains and sprains. Recently it is used to prevent post-operative pain.

Capsaicin binds to Transient Receptor Potential Vanilloid Type 1 (TRPV1) receptor. Vanilloid receptor type 1 is a member of the transient receptor potential family of ion channels, is a modestly calcium-selective ion channel located in C-fiber and Aδ sensory neurons as well as in a growing number of other sites such as the central nervous system or the bladder [Szallasi, 2001] and when activated produces desensitization or degeneration of the sensory afferent. Mice deficient of TRPV1 show impaired pain response to heat [Caterina et al., 2000]. Capsaicin is a heat activated calcium channel with a threshold to open between 37°C and 45°C, causes the channel to lower its opening threshold, thereby opening it at temperatures less than the body's temperature that is why capsaicin is linked to the sensation of heat. Weisman et al [1994] reported that topical capsaicin (0.075%) for six weeks produced a reduction in inflammatory mediators including substances P in synovial fluid of patients with rheumatoid arthritis. Botulinium toxin A suppressed the trigeminal/cervical nociceptive system (hyperalgesia and vasomotor activity) activated by intradermal injection of capsaicin to the forehead of healthy subjected [Gazerani et al., 2006]. Prolonged activation of these neurons by capsaicin depletes presynaptic substance P. There is evidence that capsaicin interacted with tetradotoxin in favor of synergism to suppress the thermal nociception [Kohane et al., 1999]. Neurons that do not contain TRPV1 are unaffected. The rationale for the topical application of capsaicin and other vanilloids in the treatment of pain is that such compounds selectively excite and subsequently desensitize nociceptive neurons. This desensitization is triggered by the activation of vanilloids receptor (TRPV1) which leads to an elevation in intracellular calcium level. The application of vanilloid agonists to the peripheral nerves provide conduction blockade. This is not associated with suppression of motor or sensory functions not related to pain as with a local anaesthetic. Fitzgerald and Woolf [1982] reported that capsaicin (1.5%) applied locally to a peripheral nerve provided inhibition of responses to noxious heat stimuli for up to 16 days, but noxious mechanical stimuli were unaffected by this treatment. Topical capsaicin preparations (0.025-0.075%) are available for human use and produces benefit in postherpetic neuralgia, diabetic neuropathy, postmastectomy pain syndrome, oral neuropathic pain, trigeminal neuralgia, tempromandibular joint disorder, cluster headache and osteoarthritis. Capsaicin is not satisfactory for chronic pain, and is often adjuvant to other approaches [Watson, 1994].

Homocapsaicin

It is a capsaicinoid and analog and congener of capsaicin in chili peppers (*Capsicum*). It accounts for about 1% of the total capsaicinoids mixture and has about half the pungency of capsaicin. It is a lipophilic colorless odorless crystalline to waxy compound.

Resiniferatoxin

Resiniferatoxin (RTX), isolated from *Euphorbia resinifera*, is a natural product in which the alkyl C-region of capsaicin is replaced with a tricyclic diterpene structurally related to those found in the phorbol esters. It is much more potent than capsaicin [Szallasi et al., 1999]. In experimental animal it produced a long standing thermal and mechanical hypoalgesia with a very wide separation between effective concentrations (0.00003-0.001%), providing an effect lasting from several hours to several weeks. Xu et al., [1997] reported that the systemic administration of RTX (0.5 mg/kg subcutaneously) caused a marked thermal hypoalgesia that started to recover after two weeks and also caused mechanical hypoalgesia, which recovered a week after the injection. Systemic injection of RTX destroys TRPV1-expressing sensory neurons and induces a long-lasting impairment of thermal nociception in adult rats [Pan et al., 2003]. Percutaneous administration of RTX to peripheral nerves can provide long-lasting suppression, not only thermal but also mechanical nociception [Kissin et al., 2002]. Resiniferatoxin-induced conduction blockade has an inherent drawback of TRPV1 agonist, the initial excitation (pain) [Kissin, 2008].

E. Neurotoxins

Cervical dystonia, also called spasmodic torticollis, is the third most common movement disorder, after Parkinson's disease and tremor, affecting approximately 125,000 people in the United States. The symptoms of cervical dystonia usually develop gradually over a period of time, with the severity of symptoms leveling off after five years. This excessive muscle activity is often painful. In one study of 170 patients, more than 90 percent of cervical dystonia patients experienced chronic pain [Zesiewicz et al., 2004]. Neurotoxins are currently used to treat this condition.

Botulinum Toxin

Botulinum toxin is a neurotoxin produced by *Clostridium botulinum,* spore-forming anaerobic bacillus. It cleaves synaptic vesicle association membrane protein (synaptobrevin) which is a component of the protein complex responsible for docking and fusion of the synaptic vesicle to the presynaptic membrane. It blocks acetylcholine release and then paralyzes the muscle for 3-4 months.

In December 1989, botulinium toxin A was approved by the US Food and Drug Administration (FDA) for the treatment of strabismus, blepharospasm, and hemifacial spasm in patients over 12 years old. Botulinium toxin A (Botox) is approved by FDA for treating severe spasm of neck muscle and severe primary axillary hyperhidrosis. Botulinium Toxin Type B (Myobloc) received FDA approval for treatment of cervical dystonia on December, 2000. The specific biological activity for (Botox) is 60 MU-Ev/ng neurotoxin, for Dysport 10 MU-Ev/ng neurotoxin, and for Myobloc/Neurobloc 5 MU-EV/ng neurotoxin. Botulinium toxin A or B indicated for cervical dystonia when all of the following criteria are met:

- There are clonic and/or tonic involuntary contractions of multiple neck muscles.
- There is sustained head torsion and/or tilt with with limited range of motion in the neck.
- Duration of the condition is greater than six months.
- Secondary causes of dystonia are excluded e.g. chronic neuroleptic syndrome, contractures or other neuro-muscular disorders.

Botulinium toxin A is effective therapy for neck muscle spasm (cervical dystonia) and myofacial neck pain (Sycha et al., 2004). Acute-onset posttraumatic cervical dystonia is poorly responded to botulinium toxin A injections [Tarsy, 1998].

Botulinium injections reduced motor end plate activity and the interference pattern of electromyography significantly but had no effect on either pain (spontaneous or referred) or pain thresholds compared with isotonic saline [Qerama et al., 2006]. The findings of Qerama et al., study are in agreement with Ojala et al., study [2006] who found in a double blind, randomized, controlled cross-over study that there was no difference between the effect of small doses of botulinium toxin A and those of the physiological saline in the treatment of myofacial pain syndrome as well as Ferrante et al [2005] who, in randomized, double blind, placebo controlled study, reported that injection of botulinium toxin A directly into trigger points did not improve cervico-thoracic myofascial pain.

Freund and Schwartz (2000) reported a significant improvement in objective of total range of neck motion and subjective pain in patients with whiplash associated disorder. The effect of botulinium toxin A persists for several weeks and neck weakness is the adverse reaction of such therapy (Bihari, 2005). Subsequent treatment is associated with no therapeutic response in 5-10% i.e. resistance due to formation of blocking antibodies (Klein, 2002). Single intramuscular injection of botulinium toxin sero B relieved the pain of cervical dystonia in patients who poorly responded to botulinium toxin A (Costa et al.,2004). Injection of botulinum toxin A into neck extensor musculature may cause rapidly progressive cervical kyphosis [Hogan et al., 2006]

Antibodies can develop after repeated use of high doses of botulinium toxin A in some individuals, making further treatment ineffective indefinitely. Because of unique mechanism of action and antigenicity of botulinium toxin A, it may be effective in patients with cervical dystonia who developed antibodies or who have not responded to botulinium toxin B. An estimated 5-15% of patients with injected serially with 79-11 Botox developed secondary non-responsiveness from the production of neutralizing antibodies. Risk factors associated with the development of neutralizing antibodies include injection of more than 200 units per session and repeated a booster injection given within one month of treatment. The new BCB 2024 Botox may have a lower potential for neutralizing antibody production because of its decreased protein load. Antibodies are produced in association with certain treatment parameters, patients'characteristics and immunological properties of the botulinium toxin preparation used [Dressler and Hallett, 2006]. For myobloc/Neurobloc, this translates into an antibody-induced therapy failure rate of 44% in patients treated for cervical dystonia whereas for BTX-A preparation this figure is approximately 5%.

F. Alpha-2 Adrenoceptor Agonists

α_2-adrenoceptor agonists are nonspecific analgesics. Although the overall response rate appears to be only fair, some patients clearly benefit. Potentially, any type of pain may be treated with these drugs. Injection of α_2-adrenoceptor agonists along axon has been suggested to improve the nerve block characteristics of local anesthetic solution through either a local vasoconstriction [Gaumann et al., 1992], a facilitation of C-fiber blockade from the local anesthetic solution [Gaumann et al., 1994] or spinal action cause by slow retrograde axonal transport or single diffusion along the nerve [Brimijoin and Helland, 1976].

Tizanidine

It is related to centrally acting skeletal muscle relaxant. It is α_2 agonist adrenergic receptor presumably reduces spasticity by increasing presynaptic inhibition of motor neurons. The effects of tizanidine are greatest on polysynaptic pathways.

It can be effective for tension headache, back pain, neuropathic pain and myofascial pain. Although clonidine has been used for refractory neuropathic pain, tizanidine tended to be better tolerated than clonidine and unlike clonidine, rarely decreased blood pressure. The sedative property of tizanidine may benefit patients with insomnia caused by severe muscle spasm [See and Ginsburg, 2008]. Tizanidine is used to relieve the spasms and increased muscle tone caused by multiple sclerosis, stroke, or brain spinal injury. It is indicated for treating muscle spasm in patients with cervical strain. Tizanidine as baclofen may have less potential for addiction.

Clonidine

The addition of clonidine to local anesthetic solution improved peripheral nerve blockade by reducing the onset time, extending postoperative analgesia and improving the efficacy of nerve block during surgery [Bernard and Macarie, 1997; Salonen et al., 1992]

In the double blind study by De Kock [1999], an infusion of clonidine 6 mg/kg/hr reduced intra-opertaive intravenous propofol and post-opertaive analgesic requirements, with only asymptomatic bradycardia. Further double-blind, placebo controlled trial by Murga et al [1994], intra-operative requirements of fentanyl is reduced by 50% and provided post-operative analgesia for hours without significant reduced blood pressure.

G. NMDA- Receptor Antagonists

There are several drugs that block NMDA receptor. All these drugs are used now to treat neuropathic pain. These drugs include: dextromethorphan, amantadine, memantine and ketamine.

Dextromethorphan

Dextromethorphan is a low-affinity, noncompetitive *N*-methyl-D-aspartate (NMDA) receptor antagonist used to treat a variety of painful conditions. It inhibits both wind-up and NMDA receptor-mediated nociceptive responses of secondary-order neurons within the spinal cord dorsal horn [Dickenson et al., 1991; Tal and Bennett, 1993].

In one placebo-controlled, double-blind, randomized crossover study, single dose (270 mg) of dextromethophan hydrobromide produced a statistically significant analgesic effect, compared with placebo, in patients with post-traumatic neuropathic pain [Carlsson et al., 2004]. In randomized, double-blind, crossover trial, oral dextromethorphan for 6 weeks had no significant analgesic effect in pain due to possible trigeminal neuropathy and anesthesia dolorosa [Gilron et al .,2000].

Amantadine

Amantadine is an NMDA receptor antagonist which may help prevent the central nervous system changes associated with chronic pain that make chronic pain difficult to treat. Amantadine was originally developed as an anti-viral medication and has been also used to treat Parkinson's disease. In experimental randomized, blinded, and placebo controlled study, Lascelles et al [2008] demonstrated that the addition of amantadine to meloxicam improved the physical activity of dogs with refractory osteoarthritic pain. It is an attractive "third man in" for patients inadequately managed on NSAIDs and tramadol or it can be teamed with an opioid alone (tramadol or oral morphine) in NSAID intolerant patients.

Memantine

Although NMDA receptors play a substantial role in central nervous system changes underlying neuropathic pain, Wiech et al [2004] found that memantine a NMDA receptor antagonist no effect on the intensity of chronic phantom limb pain.

Ketamine

Treatment options for patients with chronic persistent pain, who received narcotic analgesia, include dose escalation, opioid rotation, drug holidays, and the addition of adjuvants. Some experts advocate the use of N-MDA-receptor antagonists to combat tolerance. The effect of ketamine on neuropathic pain seems to be more potent than that of dextromethorphan [Mao, 2002]. Intravenous ketamine test may be a valuable tool in predicting subsequent response to dextromethorphan treatment in opioid-exposed patients [Cohen et al 2004]. No significant differences in the response to either ketamine or dextromethorphan treatment based on pain classification (i.e., nociceptive, neuropathic, or mixed) or placebo response [Cohen et al., 2008].

H. Muscle Relaxants

Muscle relaxants are thought to be useful in pain disorders based on the theory that pain induces spasm and spasm causes pain. Central muscle relaxants act as sedatives which most likely cause their muscle relaxant effects. They are commonly used to treat muscle spasms in the neck pain. Spasmolytics like carisoprodol, cyclobenzaprine, metaxalone and methocarbamol, are commonly prescribed for low back pain or neck pain, fibromyalgia, tension headache and myofascial pain syndrome. They are not more effective than paracetamol or non-steroidal anti-inflammatory drugs, and in fibromyalgia they are not more effective than antidepressants [Chou et al., 2007; van Tulder et al., 2003]. Centrally acting muscle relaxants are usually used in the treatment of neuropathic pain. Examples of these drugs; Gabapentin, Fosphenytoin, Tapentadol, Locasamide, Bicifadin. Fosphenytoin is a sodium channel blocker anticonvulsant showed significant analgesic effect in patients with central neuropathic pain following spinal cord injury compared to lignocain [Sang et al., 2006]. Tapentadol , a centrally acting analgesic acts by activation of mu opioid receptor and inhibit reuptake norepinephrine. Its analgesic potency is higher than corresponding tramadol but less than morphine [Tzchentke et al., 2006]. Carbamazepine is considered first-line therapy for trigeminal neuralgia. Clinical trials suggest its efficacy for treating diabetic neuropathy, but results are mixed for postherpetic neuralgia. Gabapentin is more effective than placebo at reducing diabetic neuropathy and postherpetic neuralgia-associated pain. In experimental animal model, inytrathecal gabapentin prevents the development of spinal opioid tolerance (Hansen et al., 2004). Lamotrigine shows promise for decreasing pain associated with trigeminal neuralgia.

Baclofen

It is a derivative of γ-aminobutyric acid (GABA) primarily used to treat spasticity. It is a specific GABA-B receptor agonist and its beneficial effect result from actions at spinal and supraspinal sites unrelated to GABA. Tolerance does not seem to occur to any significant degree in that baclofen retains its therapeutic antispasmodic effects even after many years of chronic use [Gaillard, 1977]. Intrathecal baclofen is used for treatment moderate or severe generalized dystonia, particularly secondary dystonia [Albright et al., 2003]. Dykstra et al [2005] reported two cases with cervical dystonia who were not responded to oral medications and became resistant to botulinum toxin A and B injections but were successfully treated with high cervical (C1-C3) continuously infused (pump implant) intrathecal baclofen. Baclofen's site of action in treating dystonia is unknown. It may be at the spinal cord level or the cortical level or both. It is capable of inhibiting both monosynaptic reflexes at the spinal level, possibly by hyperpolarization of afferent terminals, although actions at supraspinal site may also occur and contribute to its clinical effects. The analgesic effect of baclofen may be related to inhibition of neural function presynaptically by reducing calcium ion influx and thereby reducing the release of excitatory neurotransmitters in both brain and spinal cord. Also it inhibits the release of substance P in the spinal cord [Cazalets et al., 1998].

Penerai et al [1985] found that baclofen pretreatment in human prolonged the duration of fentanyl-induced analgesia from 18 to 30 minutes in patients undergoing neurosurgical anesthesia.

Cyclobenzaprine

It is a tricyclic antidepressant compound that is used clinically as a long acting muscle relaxant and analgesic. It was originally shown to be of some benefit in the management of fibromyalgia in the mid-1980s [Lautenschlager, 2000]. It shares structural and pharmacological similarities with the tricyclic antidepressants [Rao, 2002]. Its mechanism of action may be mediated by blockade of 5-HT$_2$ receptors [Rao, 2002].

It was more effective than placebo for managing neck and back pain particularly in the first four days of therapy [Browning et al., 2001]. Cyclobenzaprine alone showed significant improvements in patients with acute neck and back pain with spasm but it did not showed significant synergistic effect with ibuprofen [Childers et al., 2005]

I. Biological Drugs

The clinical uses of these drugs are so limited in cervical spine disorders and they are still under experimental and clinical investigations. They are sub-grouped into:

1. Anti tumor necrosis factor-alpha (TNF$_\alpha$)
2. Interleukin-1 (IL-1) blockers
3. Interleukin-1 (IL-1) Trap

1. Anti tumor necrosis factor-alpha (TNF$_\alpha$) e.g. etanercept, infliximab, adalimumab, certolizumab.

Tumor necrosis factor-alpha (TNF$_\alpha$) is a cytokine produced by monocytes and macrophages. It increases the migration of leucocytes to the inflammatory area. There are two types of TNF$_\alpha$ receptors found in leucocytes that respond to TNF by releasing other cytokines, and soluble TNF receptor that inactivate TNF and blunt the immune response.

Etanercept

It is a recombinant-DNA drug made by combining two proteins (a fusion protein). It links human soluble TNF-receptor to the Fc component of IgG$_1$. Etanercept mimics the inhibitory effects of naturally occurring soluble TNF receptor but has extended half-life in blood stream [Madhusudan et al., 2005]. It binds to TNF$_\alpha$ and decreases its role in disorders involving excess inflammation in humans and othe animals including autoimmune diseases such as ankylosing spondylitis [Braun et al., 2007], juvenile rheumatoid arthritis, psoriasis, psoriatic arthritis, rheumatoid arthritis. It was released for commercial use in late 1998. Experimental data showed that etanercept has a neurotoxic effect when injected into the endonerve [Wagner and Myers, 1996]. In controlled, non-randomized clinical study, patients with severe sciatica had sustained improvement, assessed by visual analogue scale for leg pain and for low back pain, after a short period of treatment with etanercept [Genevay and Singelin, 2004]. Zanella et al [2008] reported the significant long-lasting analgesic effect of a locally administered polymeric formulation of etanercept in an inflammatory neuropathic pain using unilateral chronic constriction injury of rat sciatic nerve. It did not affect the expression of CGRP neurons after nerve injury, therefore the analgesic effect of etanercept is not due to suppression of inflammatory neuropeptides [Norimoto et al., 2008]. Immediate intrathecal treatment with etanercept resulted in markedly reduced mechanical allodynia up to 4 weeks after spinal cord injury involved T13 spinal cord hemisection [Marchand et al., 2008] This finding may offer therapeutic opportunities of etanercept for treating spinal cord injury pain.

2. Interleukin-1 (IL-1) Blockers e.g. Anakinara

Interleukin-1 is a protein secreted by many cells in the body, it can trigger disease activity. Anakinara is an IL-1 receptor antagonist. It is recombinant, non glycosylated version of human IL-1 receptor antagonist. It is a biological response modifier. It is prepared from cultures of genetically modified *E coli* using recombinant DNA technology. It blocks the biological activity of naturally occurring IL-1 including inflammation and cartilage degradation associated with rheumatoid arthritis by competitively inhibiting the binding of IL-1 to the IL-1 receptor which is expressed in many tissues and organs.

3. Interleukin-1 (IL-1) Trap e.g. Rilonacept

Rilonacept prevents IL-1 from attaching to cell-surface receptors, creating a flare in disease. It was given as an orphan drug status by United States- Food and Drug administration. It is a dimeric fusion protein for the treatment of cryopyrin associated periodic syndromes including familial cold autoinflammatory syndrome and Muckle-Wells syndrome. Cryopyrin associated periodic syndrome associated syndrome is a life long, recurrent rash, fever, chills, joint pain, eye redness, eye pain and fatigue. These symptoms were triggered and exacerbated by cooling temperature, stress or exercise.

J. Adenosine

Endogenous denosine modulates the pain perception by activation the antinociceptive adenosine A_1-receptor within the central nervous system [Sawynok and Sweeney, 1989; Lee and Yaksh, 1998]. It is known that the antiallodynic effects of adenosine are mediated through the activation of spinal adenosine A_1 receptors and motor dysfunction effects are mediated through adenosine A_2 receptors at the spinal level [Lee and Yaksk, 1996]. Activation of adenosine A1 receptors at the spinal level is required for the synergistic interaction on the mechanical allodynia [Park and Jun, 2008]. Spinally administered adenosine reduces hypersensitivity in animals and humans with nerve injury, but also causes transient pain in humans and reduces tonic inhibition in spinal neurons. In rats, intrathecal administration of ATP and the P2X-receptor agonist alpha, beta-methylene-ATP produced tactile allodynia which lasted more than 1 week and it is prevented by intrathecal administration of selectiveP2X3/P2X2/3 receptor antagonist [Nakagawa et al., 2007].

The antinociceptive effects of intrathecal adenosine were seen in a model of central neuropathic pain demonstrated in a model of spinal cord ischemia [Sjölund et al 1998]. Intrathecal injection of adenosine reduced the spontaneous and evoked pain in patients with chronic neuropathic pain [Belfrage et al., 1999].

Chronic intrathecal adenosine induces hypersensitivity in normal rats and that chronic blockade of spinal adenosine A1 receptors by the A1 antagonist 8-cyclopentyl-1,3-dipropylxanthine partially prevents nerve injury-induced hypersensitivity [Martin et al., 2006]. In human being chronic use of adenosine in a pump proved to be technically problematic and not advocated to use it [Lind et al., 2007].

K. Cholinergic drugs

A major site of analgesic action of cholinergic agents is the spinal cord. Spinal cholinergic receptors have been shown to have a potent antinociceptive action. Activation of muscarinic acetylcholine receptor inhibits spinal nociceptive transmission by potentiation of GABAergic tone through M_2, M_3 and M_4 subtypes and increases the synaptic GABA release through calcium influx and voltage-gated calcium channels [Zhang et al., 2008]. It is believed that the analgesia after spinal cholinesterase inhibition by neostigmine is mediated through muscarinic, but not nicotinic cholinergic. Spinal administration of neostigmine produced a dose-dependent increase on the thermally evoked hind paw withdrawal latency in rats [Naguib andYaksh, 1994]. Systemic administration of cholinesterase inhibitors which cross the blood brain barrier have long been known to produce analgesia and enhance analgesia from opiates. Spinal injection of cholinergic agonists results in analgesia to experimental, acute postoperative, and chronic pain which primarily reflects muscarinic receptor activation [Eisenach,1990]. In rats, both bethanechol and neostigmine reduced mechanical hyperalgesia [Prado and Dias, 2008].

L. Cannabinoids

Systemic or spinal administration of Δ^9-tetrahydrocannabinol (THC) and synthetic cannabinoids have antinociceptive and antihyperalgesic effects in a variety of animal models of acute and inflammatory pain [Pertwee, 2001; Iversen and Chapman, 2002]. The antinociceptive effects of THC or anandamide are mediated via CB_1-receptors (also known CNR1) and vanilloid (VR_1) receptor [DiMarzo et al., 2001]. THC and morphine potentiation was observed in tests of acute pain [Fuentes et al., 1999] and chronic inflammatory pain [Welch and Stevens, 1992]. There is evidence that supraspinal CB_2 (also known CNR2) receptors in the thalamus may contribute to the modulation of neuropathic pain responses [Jhaveri et al, 2008]. Cannabinoid agonists are already used clinically as antiemetic or to stimulate appetite. Potential therapeutic uses of cannabinoid receptor agonists include the management of multiple sclerosis, spinal cord injury, pain, inflammatory disorders, glaucoma, bronchial asthma and cancer [Singh and Budhiraja, 2006].

M. Non-Patch Type Topical Pain Relievers

Topical pain relieving drugs include preparations applied to the skin as cream, ointment, gel spray or patch. Topical drugs reduce the subcutaneous inflammation and soothe nerve pain. Topical analgesics differ from transdermal delivery systems, that is introduced in 1980, in that the latter's goal is to deliver systemic rather than local effects. Topical medicine used to treat pain associated with osteoarthritis, rheumatoid arthritis, neck or low back strain, whiplash, muscle inflammation and spasms and some types of nerve pain. The advantages of topical medicine include: its application is easy and controllable, the onset of symptoms relief is usually faster than oral preparations, also a steady rate and longer duration of symptom relief were observed with topical medicine,a smaller amount may be needed and topical medicine is not subjected to fast pass metabolism. The Disadvantages of topical medicine include certain types of back and neck pain will not respond to topical treatment and skin hypersensitivity reactions may occur. Topical Analgesia include: Lidocaine (5%), Capsaicin (0.025-0.75%), Resiniferatoxin (0.00003-0.001%), Doxepin (3.3%), Amitriptyline (2%) and Ketamine (1%). They are effective moderately in peripheral neuropathic pain with allodynia and should consider as a therapeutic option but should be evaluated on an individual basis (Besson et al., 2008).

Ketamine

Lynche et al (2005a andb) demonstrated the effectiveness of 1% ketamine or 2% amitryptiline or 2% amitriptyline-1% ketamine combined in reducing the pain intensity assessed by 11 point numerical scale in neuropathic patients in randomized double blind placebo control and open labeled studies. In clinical reports, topical ketamine was reported to produce analgesia in case studies involving neuropathic and cancer pain [Crowley, 1998; Wood, 2000]. In experimental animal model ketamine produced an antihyperalgesic but not an analgesic action and produced no analgesia [Oatway et al., 2003]. Ketamine inhibits NMDA-receptors in neuronal preparations, and this could lead to the antihyperalgesic action [Hirota and Lambert 1996].

It is antihyperalgesic in acute inflammatory pain [Warncke et al., 1997] provides some direct analgesia [Pederson et al., 1998], inhibits sympathetically maintained pain [Crowley et al., 1998], but has no analgesic effects on capsaicin-induced hyperalgesia [Gottrup et al., 2000, 2004]

Amitriptyline

Ho et al (2008) found that 5% amitriptyline was ineffective in reducing pain intensity using a 0 to 100 mm visual analog scale in patients with neuropathic pain (postsurgical neuropathic pain, postherpetic neuralgia, or diabetic neuropathy with allodynia or hyperalgesia). There is evidence that trans-cutaneous amitriptyline solution has a differential effect on different fiber structures. It induced a mild and short-lasting increase of the tactile and mechanical nociceptive thresholds and it significantly decreased cold and heat thresholds [Dualé et al., 2008].

Amitriptyline produced both an antihyperalgesic and an analgesic action in the sensitized paw rat and produced analgesia in the nonsensitized paw rat [Oatway et al., 2003].

Amitriptyline like ketamine inhibits NMDA-receptors in neuronal preparations, and this could lead to the antihyperalgesic action [Reynolds and Miller, 1988].

Doxepin

Topical doxepin, a tricyclic antidepressant, produced analgesia in placebo-controlled trials of neuropathic pain [McCleane, 2000 a, b]. In the first study, doxepin (5%) was applied for 4 weeks, and produced significant analgesia in the last 10 days of treatment, but not in the 1st week. In the larger study, topical doxepin (3.3%) was compared with topical capsaicin (0.025%) and a combination of doxepin with capsaicin. Significant reductions in overall pain scores were observed for all treatment groups from week 2 to 4, but the combination group had a faster onset of action with analgesia at 1 week. A burning discomfort after cream application was noted by 81% in the capsaicin group, 61% in the doxepin/capsaicin group, and 17% in the doxepin group. Antidepressants exhibit promise as a useful class of agents to be used as analgesics following topical application and other methods of local delivery.

N. Spinal injections

Intrathecal analgesia has emerged as a key therapeutic option for pain relief for patients who have failed other treatment avenues as well as patients with adequate analgesia on high dose entral or parentral therapy but with unacceptable side effects. Leonard Corning is credited with neuraxial administration of local anesthetic in 1885, and morphine may have been administered spinally as early as 1901[Matsuki, 1983].

Facet Joint Injection

The prevalence of facet joint pain is 55% in chronic cervical spinal pain [Manchikanti et al., 2004b]. Cervical facet pain is not characterized as easily as lumbar facet pain. It can occur with a variety of symptoms depending on the cervical level. Headache, neck pain spasm and general or focal neck pain can originate from the facet pain. This pain is typically worse when the patients extend or turn their neck. The upper cervical facets can often cause occipital headache. There are two methods of facet joint injection: the direct posterior and posterior-lateral approaches. A total amount of injected fluid is not usually more than 1.5 milliliter in the cervical spine (the capacity of a cervical facet joint is 0.5-1 milliliter). Common mixture is betamethasone, triamcinolone acetonide with bupivacaine, lidocaine. The optimal injection is made directly into the joint space. Pain relief following a precise intra-articular injection confirms the facet joint the source of pain. Long term relief (up to 6 months) can be obtained with steroids in 30-50% of patients. The most common causes that required facet joint injections are: degenerative disease, synovitis (overt or radiologically occult), post laminectomy syndrome and non radicular pain. Although facet joint injections rarely carried complications but they may include: bleeding, infection, allergic reactions, false negative response and accidental injection into vertebral artery or radicular branches can be dangerous. Some patients experience transient adverse effects (e.g. insomnia, nightmares) from the steroids and life-threatening idiopathic reaction to any medication was also observed. Facet joint injection is contraindicated in patients with history of allergy, coagulopathy, and severe foraminal stenosis because swelling of the joint may temporarily result in exacerbation of the patient's symptoms. Intra cervical zygapophyseal joints injections with the mixture of lidocaine [0.5 ml of 1%] and triamcinolone [5 mg] of patients with cervical zygapophyseal joint pain, were diagnosed originally as myofascial pain syndrome (MPS), cervical herniated nucleus pulposus (HNP), and whiplash-associated disorders (WAD) resulted in the immediate reduction of pain and the analgesic effect lasted longer in cervical HNP than MPS or WAD [Kim et al.,2005].

Selective Nerve Block, Transforaminal Epidural Injection

Epidural injections for managing chronic pain are one of the most commonly performed interventions in the United States [Manchikanti et al., 2006]. Epidural steroid injections via a transforaminal approach, given the extremely small possibility for catastrophic complications that has been described. It is indicated in patients with radicular pain, with or without an axial component, originating from the cervical spine [Bush et al., 1996; Slipman et al., 2000]. It acts by suppression of the inflammatory response surrounding the targeted nerve roots [Molloy et al., 2005]. The complications of cervical transforaminal epidural steroid injection included acute infarction involving the cervical spine and extending to the cervicomedullary junction [Muro et al., 2007]. Scanlen et al [2007] demonstrated a significant risk (78 out of

1340 cases) of serious neurologic injury and mortality rate (~1%) after cervical transforaminal epidural steroid injections.

Intrathecal Pump

Morphine is the only opioid drug approved by the FDA for intreathecal delivary to treat chronic pain. Opioids administered neuraxially, act at receptors in the substantia gelatinosa of the spinal cord dorsal horn to yield dose-dependent analgesia [Pert and Snyder, 1973; Terenius, 1973]. Systemically administered morphine leads to an opioid-induced increase in spinal acetylcholine, and the opioid-induced spinal acetylcholine via activation of the spinal cholinergic system contributes to opioid-mediated antinociception [Nallu and Radhakrishnan, 2007]. Intrathecal (morphine) pump is used for chronic pain, cancer pain and for chronic spasticity. It increases pain relief in patients with severe pain and improves the quality of life and allows the patients to participate more fully in daily activities. A small pump is surgically placed under the skin of the abdomen to deliver medication directly into the area surrounded the spinal area via catheter. Long-term intrathecal opioid infusions can be effective in treatment of neuropathic pain but might require higher infusion doses [Anderson and Burchiel, 1999; Hassenbusch et al., 1995]. Hydromorphone, a semisynthetic hydrogenated ketone of morphine, is a more potent and faster-acting analgesic than morphine due to its greater lipophilic properties. Analgesic response was improved by a least 25% in patients with chronic nonmalignant pain who were switched from intraspinal morphine to hydromorphone because of poor pain relief [Anderson et al., 2001], and also the adverse reactions were improved. Intrathecal morphine and intrathecal hydromorphone (in a dose 20% of that of morphine) induce an equi-analgesic response [Ruan, 2007].

Sympathetic or Somatic Nerve Block

The occipital pain and headache of cervical arthritis also often respond to injection of 2 to 3 ml of long-acting anesthetic into the greater and lesser occipital nerves at the sites where they pierce the trapezius muscle [Carron, 1978].

Several drugs are currently used like steroids, local anaesthetics, opiods, muscle relaxants and α_2 adrenoceptor agonists.

Corticoteroids

It is believed that epidural administration of corticosteroids and/or local anesthetic altered or interrupted the nociceptive input, reflex mechanisms of the afferent fibers, self sustaining activity of the neurons, and the pattern of central neuronal activities. Corticosteroids reduce inflammation by inhibiting either the synthesis or release of a number of proinflammatory mediators and by causing a reversible local anaesthetic effect [Lundin et al., 2005; Lee et al., 1998]. Injections of corticosteroids into or adjacent to the spinal canal is performed on a regular basis in the United States. The use of methylprednisolone administration in the treatment of acute spinal cord injury is not proven as a standard of care, nor can it be considered a recommended treatment because its efficacy and impact is weak [John Hurlebert, 2000].

However, epidural steroids injections are used for herniated disc, sciatica, radiculopathy, spinal stenosis. Cervical epidural steroid injection have been used to treat the following conditions: pain associated with acute disc herniation and radiculopathy, postlaminectomy cervical pain, cervical strain syndromes with associated myofascial pain, and postherpetic neuralgia. Rowlingson and Kirschenbaum [1986] described significant reduction in upper extremity pain after cervical epidural steroid injections, and other studies identified radicular pain relief via interlaminar and transforaminal approaches. Transforaminal cervical epidural steroids injections provide long term pain relief in patients with neck pain and radiculopathy [Bush and Hillier, 1996] and cervical disc surgery [Lin et al., 2006; Kolstad et al; 2005]. The fact that corticosteroids differ significantly in microscopic size has become an important consideration because of an awareness that the larger a particle is, the greater are its chances of occluding a blood vessel should the compound be inadvertently injected vascularly. A study that analyzed the microscopic size of the aforementioned corticosteroids found the following:

Dexamethasone - Particles were 5-10 times smaller than red blood cells, contained few particles, and showed no aggregation.

Triamcinolone - Particles varied greatly in size, were densely packed, and formed extensive aggregations. It provides a sustained anti-inflammatory effect.

Betamethasone - Particles varied greatly in size, were densely packed, and formed extensive aggregations. It provides rapid onset and extended anti-inflammatory activity. The dose for intralaminar approach is 12-18 mg and half of this dose for transforaminal approach.

Methylprednisolone particles were relatively uniform in size, smaller than red blood cells, and densely packed and did not form very many aggregations. It provides a sustained anti-inflammatory effect. Because injected methylprednisolone has been reported to remain in situ for approximately 2 weeks, the clinician should expect to wait 2 weeks after the injection to assess the patient's response and to administer a repeat injection. The dose for intralaminar approach is 80-120 mg and half of this dose for transforaminal approach.

In cervical epidural injections, a total of 3-5 mL may be used for epidural steroid injections employing the interlaminar approach. However, in transforaminal approach, clinicians generally use a total volume of only about 1.5 mL. Neuraxial steroid injections are generally considered to be safe in the U.S. The following complications of steroid injections are reported:

(a) Direct spinal injury. Damage to the spinal cord at the level of the cervical spine will often result in greater impairment than will damage at the lumbar levels and may precipitate respiratory arrest at higher cervical levels. There is evidence that cervical epidural injection is rarely complicated by spinal cord injury and neurological deficit [Hodges et al., 1998; Brouwers et al., 2001]. The possible mechanism of injury is embolization of the spinal cord due to injection of steroid into a radicular artery Baker et al 2003].
(b) Hematoma. Epidural hematoma occurs in 0.01-0.02% of performed procedures.
(c) Infection
(d) Inflammatory complications
(e) Others: anterior cord syndrome, presumably resulting from the injection of particulate into the artery of Adamkiewicz

Absolute contraindications for epidural steroid injections include the following:

(a) Systemic infection or local infection at the site of a planned injection
(b) Bleeding disorder or fully anticoagulated (for example, on a fully "therapeutic" dose of coumadin, heparin).
(c) History of significant allergic reactions to injected solutions (eg, contrast, anesthetic, corticosteroid)
(d) Acute spinal cord compression
(e) Patient refusal to proceed with the injection procedure

Local Anaesthetics (Bupivacaine, Lidocaine)

Local anaesthetics interrupt the spine-spasm cycle and reverberating nociceptor transmission. Intrathecal local anesthetics are commonly used in combination with opioids. Intrathecal combinations of local anesthetics and opioids provided synergistic analgesic effects and decreased opioid side effects [van Dongen et al., 1999; Krames, 1993]. On the other hand a multicenter, double-blind randomized study found that the addition of bupivacaine did not provide better pain relief than opioids alone [Mironer et al., 2002].

Bupivaciane should not be used in place of lidocaine for needle procedures in the cervical spine. With inadvertent intrathecal injection, respiratory comprise may be prolonged due to bupivacaine's longer duration of action.

α_2 *Adrenoceptor Agonists*

α_2-adrenergic receptors play a key role in analgesic effects mediated at peripheral, spinal and brain stem sites. It hyperpolarizes the cell by increasing potassium conductance through Gi coupled K-channels on post synaptic neurons [Wallace andYaksh, 2000]. Also it activates spinal cholinergic neurons which may potentiate its analgesic effect. Clonidine is the only FDA-approved α_2-adrenoceptor agonist for intrathecal use. Intrathecal clonidine has been reported to provide significant analgesia alone or in combination with opioids for neuropathic pain, cancer pain, or complex regional pain syndrome [Ackerman et al., 2003; Uhle et al., 2000]. Siddall et al [2000] assessed the efficacy of intrathecal morphine or clonidine, alone or combined for up to 6 days, in 15 patients with central pain secondary to spinal cord injury. They found the combination of clonidine and morphine provided significantly better pain relief than saline (37% vs. 0% reduction) or either drug alone (20% reduction for morphine, 17% decrease for clonidine).

Ziconotide

It is the synthetic equivalent of ω-conopeptide MV1A, a 25-amino-acid polybasic peptide present in the venom of conus magus, a marine snail [Olivera et al., 1985]. It produces potent antinoceptive effect by selectively binding to N-type voltage-selective calcium channels [Olivera et al., 1987; Miljanich and Ramachandran, 1995] on neuronal soma, dendrites, dendritic shafts and axon terminals, thus blocking neurotransmission from primary nociceptive afferents. Intrathecal ziconotide provided clinically and statistically significant analgesia in patients with pain from cancer or acquired immune deficiency syndrome [Staats et al., 2004].

Baclofen

Baclofen is a GABA-B agonist that has been used for muscle spasms, spasticity, and neuropathic pain. Baclofen is a racemic mixture with L-baclofen being the active form.

Intrathecal baclofen infusions have been used to treat spasticity since the mid-1980s and intrathecal baclofen administration via an implanted device is approved by the Food and Drug Administration (FDA) for this indication. Intrathecal baclofen has been proven in reducing spasticity and dystonia associated with complex regional pain syndrome without any adverse effect [Taricco et al., 2006; van Hilten et al., 2000] but less effective in reducing neuropathic pain [Loubser and Akman, 1996].

Intrathecal Cocktails

Morphine sulfate combined with bupivacaine hydrochloride and clonidine hydrochloride incubated in implantable pumps at 37°C for 90 days remained stable with more than 96% of the original concentration intact. Combinations of morphine or hydromorphone with bupivacaine have been recognized to be stable [Hildebrand et al., 2001; Classen et al., 2004] but morphine and hydromorphone facilitate ziconotide degradation. A ziconotide/ clonidine/ morphine admixture was 70% stable for 20 days while Ziconotide/ baclofen admixtures are 80% stable over 30 days.

IV. ANTIMICROBIALS

Spinal infection can occur in vertebral bone, intervertebral disc space, epidural or intradural space within the spinal canal, and adjacent soft tissues. The most commonly isolated pathogen in 50% of bone infections is *Staphylococcus aureus* [Berbari et al., 2005]. Other microorganisms that have been implicated in bone infections include gram-positive microbes, such as *Streptococci* and *Enterococci*. Gram-negative bacteria such as *Enterobacteriaceae, Pseudomonas*, and anaerobic species are less frequently associated with bone infections [Lew and Waldvogel, 1997]. The pharmacokinetic characteristics of the antimicrobial molecule (including water or lipid soluble drug, molecular size, pH of drug, partition coefficient of drug, and protein binding) and the vascular integrity of bone are the most important factors that determined the drug bone penetration. Limited numbers of antimicrobials fulfill the above criteria and are useful in treatment of spinal infections.

Single dose of piperacillin-tazobactam produced concentrations in the cancellous and cortical bone that were sufficient to assure antibacterial activity [Incavo et al., 1994]. Successful treatment of cervical spinal epidural abscess was reported with piperacillin [Moriya et al., 2005]. Ticarcillin-clavulanate achieved high bone concentrations after a single 5.2 g bolus dose. Spontaneous pseudomonas osteomyelitis of spine was successfully managed with ticarcillin and tobramycin [Breit and Nade, 1987]. Ceftriaxone and cefamandole concentrations in the bone exceeded the minimum inhibitory concentration for susceptible staphylococcal pathogens [Lovering et al., 2001]. Similarly, cefazolin, a first-generation cephalosporin with excellent activity against *S aureus*, was found to achieve bone tissue levels above minimum inhibitory concentrations for susceptible gram-positive organisms [Fass et al., 1978; Mader et al., 1989]. The mean synovial fluid concentration of cefoxitin obtained approximately half an hour after administration was >100% compared to the mean serum concentration obtained simultaneously [Schurman et al., 1982]. Meropenem effectively penetrated bone and joint tissue [Sano et al., 1993]. Rifampin is an effective adjunctive agent in treatment of staphylococcal infections. Cluzel et al. [1984] reported that cancellous bone concentrations of rifampin were greater than the minimum inhibitory concentration of *S aureus* strains up until 12 hours after a dose of 600 mg. Fluoroquinolones are attractive agents in the treatment of bone infections due to their broad antimicrobial activity and patient tolerability. A study investigating the penetration of levofloxacin into cortical and cancellous bone tissue and the synovial fluid concluded that the penetration as 100%, 50%, and 120% respectively [Rimmelé et al., 2004]. Single moxifloxacin dose 400 mg orally either 2 or 4 hours preoperatively achieved drug concentrations in the cancellous and cortical bone exceeding the minimum inhibitory concentrations for most pathogens [Malincarne et al., 2006]. Clindamycin has broad activity against gram-positive organisms such as streptococci and staphylococci and reasonably broad coverage of anaerobic bacteria. The concentration of clindamycin in infected bone was above the minimum inhibitory concentrations for susceptible *S aureus* [Nicholas et al., 1975]. Metronidazole may be a useful adjunctive agent in polymicrobial bone infections. Its concentration in human bone is not well-defined. Macleod et al. [1986] investigated the penetration of aztreonam into synovial fluid and bone and found excellent tissue levels. Linezolid is a synthetic oxazolidinone antimicrobial agent with broad gram-positive activity including MRSA and methicillin-resistant *Staphylococcus epidermidis* (MRSE) [Bassetti et al., 2005]. The penetration of linezolid into bone was rapid, with a mean concentration of 9.1 mg/L 10 minutes after infusion 600 mg of the drug. The concentration of drug in the bone when compared with simultaneous blood concentrations was 51% at 10 minutes, 60% at 20 minutes, and 47% at 30 minutes [Lovering et al., 2002]. Linezolid concentration achieved in the tissue surrounding the bone was twice the minimum inhibitory concentration of the offending pathogens [Kutscha-Lissberg et al., 2003]. The vancomycin levels in bones were higher than the minimum inhibitory concentration for susceptible staphylococci following single prophylactic intravenous dose (15 mg/kg) [Graziani et al., 1988].

In spinal infections, antimicrobials are clinically indicated for discitis, osteomyelitis and epidural abscess.

Discitis

Discitis, an inflammation of the intervertebral disc, is generally attributable to *Staphylococcus aureus* and rarely *Staphylococcus epidermidis*, *Kingella kingae*, *Enterobacteriaciae*, and *Streptococcus pneumoniae*. Cervical discitis may be much more neurologically compromising due to anatomical particularities. Cottle and Riordan [2008] recommended that unless the patient is severely unwell antimicrobial therapy should be delayed until a microbiological diagnosis is established and tentative recommendations for antimicrobial therapy can be made based on theoretical considerations. It is still not known which antibiotics are able to penetrate the intervertebral disc effectively. Antibiotic use in discitis (in children) is controversial because the course of the disease appears to be benign [Cousins et al., 1992; Ryöppy et al., 1993; Wenger et al., 1978]. Ceftriaxone is recommended in children 3 years of age or younger because of the possibility of infection by *Haemophilus influenzae*. Postoperative disc space infection was prevented with a single prophylactic dose of a first-generation cephalosporin [Osti, 1990]. Tai et al. [2002] found that cefuroxime does not diffuse into human intervertebral discs as readily as gentamicin because the later is positively charged. There is considerable evidence to suggest that the charge on antibiotics, because of their ionisable groups, is important in determining their ability to diffuse into the disc [Rhoten et al., 1995; Scuderi et al., 1993]. In brief the following drugs penetrate the disc despite of their charge: cefazolin, ceftriaxone, cefuroxime, tobramycin, gentamycin, vancomycin, teicoplanin and clindamycin. Natural or semisynthetic aminopenicillin not penetrate the intervertebral disc.

Brook [2001] reported two cases of septic discitis, one case due to *Peptostreptococcus magnus* treated with penicillin (intravenously) followed by oral ampicillin and the other showed fusiform Gram-negative bacilli with light growth *Fusobacterium nucleat*um treated with clindamycin. Vancomycin is effective against methicillin resistant staphylococcus aureus (MRSA) infections but it is less effective in treatment septic discitis due to MRSA [Al-Nammari et al., 2007]. In MRSA discitis animal model, vancomycin was superior to linezolid with a short treatment course [Conaughty et al., 2006]. The cure was achieved with long-term antimicrobial specific therapy with quinupristin-dalfopristin (50 days) and linezolid (100 days) in a case report with severe, chronic polymicrobial spine infection with epidural abscess and liquoral fistula due to multidrug-resistant organisms [Marroni et al., 2006]. A case report of cervical discitis, osteomyelitis, and epidural collection was cured with extended course of temocillin [Barton et al., 2008]. Spondylodiscitis with epidural abscess was reported to be successfully managed with ceftriaxone combined with cloxacillin [Lott-Duarte et al., 2008].

Pyogenic Osteomyleitis of the Cervical Spine

The large diameter of the cervical spinal cord relative to the spinal canal and the significant range of motion of the cervical spine make cervical osteomyelitis a unique entity. Hippocrates was the first to describe osteomyelitis of the spine in 400 BCE [cited from Dimar et al, 2004]. Establishing the diagnosis of cervical osteomyelitis in a timely fashion is critical to prevent catastrophic neurological injury [Dimar et al., 2004; Mc Henry et al., 2002]. Vertebral osteomyelitis of cervical spine accounts approximately 1-10% of all bone infections [Malawski and Lukawski, 1991; Schimmer et al., 2002]. The predominant organism in almost all studies is *Staphylococcus aureus,* accounting for approximately 40 to 80% of all spinal infections [Jensen et al., 1997]. Gram-positive organisms such as *S. epidermidis* and *Streptococcus* species are the second most common ones [Hadjipavlou et al., 2000]. Gram-negative bacteria such as *Escherichia coli,Diphtheroids, Pseudomonas, Salmonella* and *Proteus* species are also reported [Sapico et al., 1996] (Table 1). Polymicrobial infections and negative cultures are found in approximately 20% of patients [Sapico and Montgomerie, 1979, Sapico, 1996]. Blood cultures are positive in only approximately 20 to 60% of patients with spinal infection [Currier, 1998]. Mycobacterial or fungal infections should be considered in patients in whom results of cultures are persistently negative despite repeated tissue samples [Tandon and Vollmer, 2004]. Patients with overt signs of sepsis should be treated with intravenous broad-spectrum antibiotic drugs as soon as tissue is obtained for culture. Antibiotic therapy can then be tailored according to the culture and sensitivity results. Intravenous antibiotic drugs should be administered for 6 to 8 weeks, followed by a 6-week course of oral antibiotics until the infection is cured. Treatment with less than 4 weeks of antibiotic therapy is associated with a 25% relapse rate [Eismont et al., 1983; Sapico and Montgomerie, 1979; Sapico, 1996].The ESR can be expected to decrease to one half to two thirds of pretreatment levels on successful treatment [Sapico and Montgomerie, 1979; Sapico, 1996].

Epidural Abscess

Spinal epidural abscess has an estimated incidence rate of 0.2-2.8 cases per 10,000 per year with peak incidence occurring in people who are in their 60s and 70s. The most common causative agent is *staphylococcus aureus* [Martin and Yuan, 1996]. Spinal procedures (including spinal anesthesia, spinal surgery) or trauma, intravenous drug abuse, HIV infections, diabetes mellitus, alcoholism and malignancies are predisposing causes of spinal epidural abscess [Bartontini et al., 1996; Baker et al., 1975; Danner and Hartman, 1987]. The mainstay of treatment is surgical decompression. Non surgical treatment is indicated in patients with minimal neurological deficit or are poor surgical candidates [Manfredi et al., 1998]. High doses cefazolin/clindamycin combination is highly effective for patients with epidural abscess [de Goeij et al., 2008; Solomou et al., 2004; Walters et al., 2006].

V. COMPLEMENTARY/ALTERNATIVE ANALGESIA

Complementary/alternative medicine (CAM) has been defined as, "diagnosis, treatment and/or prevention that complements mainstream medicine by contributing to a common whole, by satisfying a demand not met by orthodoxy or by diversifying the conceptual frameworks of medicine [Ernst et al., 2001].

Many different CAM modalities are used to treat pain; amongst the most popular are:

Acupuncture
Trigger points
Mind-body therapy
Magnet therapy
Prolotherapy
Exercise
Spinal manipulation
Herbal preparations
Nutritional supplements

Acupuncture

It is believed that the analgesic effect of acupuncture is related to the stimulation of endorphins, serotonin, and noradrenaline secretion in the central nervous system, or release of vasodilators such as histamine (which modulate the vascular tone) or closing the gates of nerve fibers that result in pain perception. Conflicting results were reported about the effectiveness of acupuncture in neck pain. The outcomes of 14 randomized controlled trials were equally balanced between positive and negative. Acupuncture was superior to waiting-list in one study, and either equal or superior to physiotherapy in three studies, it was not superior to indistinguishable sham control in four out of five studies and five out eight high-quality trials were negative [White and Ernst,1999]. There is evidence that acupuncture needles placed in non acupuncture points lead to pain reduction because of stimulation of endorphin release via a mechanism called diffuse noxious inhibitory control [LeBars et al., 1979]. Acupuncture and other forms of acustimulation are effective in the short-term management of neck pain [Wang et al., 2008]. The success rate was higher in patients with a short duration of chronic neck pain [Blossfeldt, 2004].

Acupuncture may facilitate and/or enhance physiotherapy performance in musculoskeletal rehabilitation for tension neck syndrome in term of improving pain intensity, muscle tension, the neck disability index, and the cranio-cervical flexion test for isometric neck muscle strength [França et al., 2008]. The efficacy of acupuncture is approximated that of 0.5% lidocaine injection of trigger points in improving pain scores, range of neck movement, pressure pain intensity and depression in elderly patients with myofascial pain syndrome [Ga et al., 2007].

Trigger point acupuncture compared with standard acupuncture is significantly reduced the pain intensity and improved quality of life in patients with non radiated chronic neck pain with normal neurological examination [Itoh et al., 2007]. Guo et al [2007] found that abdominal acupuncture can significantly reduce the neck pain of the patient caused by cervical spondylosis as the traditional acupuncture.

Trigger Points

They are discrete, hyperirritable foci usually located within a taut band of skeletal muscle [Simons et al., 2002]. Pressure applied to these points produce a characteristic referred pain, tenderness and autonomic phenomena. They are an essential defining part of the myofascial pain syndrome, in which widespread or regional muscular pain is a cause of musculoskeletal dysfunction [Gerwin, 2002]. Trigger points are reported to occur more frequently in cases of mechanical neck pain than in matched controls [de Las Penas et al., 2007]. There are two types of trigger points; active and lantent.

Active trigger point that defined as one with spontaneous pain, or pain in response to movement. It is tender on palpation, and may present with a referral pattern of pain, not at the site of the trigger point origin e.g. fibromyalgia [Simons, 1986] and neck pain [Sist et al., 1999]. Rosomoff's team demonstrated that 100% of neck pain sufferers possessed the presence of trigger points and almost 53% of them had non-dermatomal referral [Rosomoff et al., 1989].

Latent trigger point is a sensitive spot that causes pain or discomfort only in response to compression. The pathogenesis of trigger points may be due to decrease in the pain pressure threshold [Fischer, 1986], or release of inflammatory mediators e.g. prostaglandins, bradykinin, serotonin or trauma [Alvarez and Rockwell, 2002]. Manual therapy [Hong et al., 1993], chiropractic treatment [Hsieh and Hong, 1990], electric therapy [Hsueh et al., 1997], local anaesthetic [McMillan et al., 1997] and active therapy [Hanten et al., 2000] have all been claimed to provide relief of trigger point sensitivity.

It is postulated that massage and myofascial release aim to increase local circulation, improve mobility and relieve subcutaneous tightness. Neuro Emotional Technique (NET) was administered to provide participants with a mind/body based treatment to relieve the sensitivity of trigger points associated with their chronic neck pain.

This technique significantly relieved pain sensitivity of trigger points presenting in a a cohort of chronic neck pain sufferers [Bablis et al., 2008]. The visual analog scale significantly decreased in sensitivity as well as pressure algometer readings significantly increased after a single NET treatment.

Mind-Body Therapy

It is behavioral, psychological, social, and spiritual approaches to medicine not commonly used. It includes: mediation, imagery, biofeedback, relaxation and hypnosis. This therapy may be effective in patients who have had rheumatoid arthritis for a short time [Astin et al., 2002]. Mindfulness meditation may be an effective strategy for helping chronic pain patients who cope more effectively with their conditions [Kabat-Zinn et al., 1985, 1987].

Magnet Therapy

Magnets may also be perceived as a more natural and less harmful alternative to analgesic compounds. It involves the application of magnetic materials on or very close to the skin over prolonged periods of time. This encompasses a wide range of interventions involving different types of devices, different strength magnetic fields and different modes of administration [Hinman, 2002]. Magnet therapy now appears to be one of the most widely used form of CAM for the management of chronic pain associated with musculoskeletal disorders such as rheumatoid arthritis. Despite the popularity of using magnets for healing pain, there is a lack of scientific evidence to prove magnets have any therapeutic benefit. Several theories were claimed, not scientifically supported, the mechanism of magnet therapy for pain heeling. These are:

1. Restoration of cellular magnetic balance.
2. Migration of calcium ions is accelerated to help heal bones and nerve tissues.
3. Circulation is enhanced since biomagnets are attracted to the iron in blood and this increase in blood flow helps healing.
4. Biomagnets have a positive effect on the pH balance of cells.
5. Hormone production is influenced by biomagnet use.

Several studies described the site, magnet support device and frequency and duration of static magnetic field (SMF) therapy but most studies failed to provide enough detail about SMF dosage to permit protocol replication by other investigators [Colbert et al., 2007].

Prolotherapy or Proliferative Injection Therapy or Regenerative Injection Therapy

Historically, the use of prolotherapy dates back to Hippocrates who treated dislocated shoulders of soldiers on the battlefields with red-hot needle cautery to stabilize the joint.

Hackett defined prolotherapy as "the rehabilitation of an incompetent structure [ligament or tendon] by the generation of new cellular tissue," and concluded that "a joint is only as strong as its weakest ligament"[Hackett et al., 1992]. Prolotherapy is a method of injection treatment designed to stimulate healing. It involves injecting an otherwise non-pharmacological and non-active irritant solution into the body, generally in the region of tendons or ligaments for the purpose of strengthening weakened connective tissue and alleviating musculoskeletal pain. This treatment is used for musculoskeletal pain which has gone on longer than 8 weeks such as low back and neck pain, chronic sprains and/or strains, whiplash injuries, tennis and golfer's elbow, knee, ankle, shoulder or other joint pain, chronic tendonitis/ tendonosis, and musculoskeletal pain related to osteoarthritis. It is based on the premise that chronic musculoskeletal pain is due to inadequate repair of fibrous connective tissue, resulting in ligament and tendon weakness or laxity [Leadbetter, 1994; Frank et al., 1985]. The injection is given into joint capsules or where tendon connects to bone. Many points may require injections. The Injected solution causes the body to heal itself through the process of inflammation and repair. Prolotherapy treatment sessions are generally given every two to six weeks. Many solutions are used, including dextrose, lidocaine (a commonly used local anesthetic) procaine, phenol (an alcohol), glycerine, or cod liver oil extract. The most common proliferant used in prolotherapy injections is hypertonic dextrose, 12.5% to 25%, with 15% being the most used. Once the cell fluid is able to dilute the dextrose, the inflammation ceases but growth factor activation continues [Reeves, 1995].

Local injection causes temporary, low grade inflammation at the site of ligament or tendon weakness (fibroosseous junction) leads to migration and activation the fibroblasts which synthesize precursors to mature collagen, and thereby reinforcing connective tissue [Reeves, 2000]. This inflammatory stimulus raises the level of growth factors to resume or initiate a new connective tissue repair sequence to complete one which had prematurely aborted or never started. Hackett reported that 82% of patients with low back pain, treated with dextrose or saline injections, considered themselves cured over periods ranging up to 12 years of follow-up [Hackett, 1959]. A series of injections of dextrose solution injected into the neck improved pain symptoms and quality of life in chronic neck pain suffers [Hauser and Hauser, 2007]. Intraarticular regeneration injection therapy improved pain and function in patients with chronic whiplash related neck pain that failed other conservative and interventional procedures [Hooper et al., 2007]. Patients were treated with intraarticular prolotherapy by placing 0.5 - 1mL of 20% dextrose solution (D50W with 1% lidocaine) into each zygapophysial joint. Dagenais et al [2007] reviewed high quality studies with a total of 366 participants with chronic low-back pain managed with prolotherapy and other co-interventions and found that prolotherapy alone was not effective therapy but may improve pain when it combined with spinal manipulation, exercise, and other co-interventions. Over 99 percent of 10,000 prolotherapy cases, found relief from their chronic pain [Hauser, 1999]. Prolotherapy is contraindicated in infections, immunodeficiency conditions, acute gout, rheumatoid arthritis, cervical stenosis, and current use of narcotics, steroids and nonsteroidal anti-inflammatory drugs. The most common risk of such therapy is bruising around the injected area. Pain after treatment, infection, and allergy are also reported.

Exercise

Exercise interventions are deemed for the effective management of patients with neck pain. Janda [1994] suggested that the cervical flexor muscles become dysfunctional in the presence of neck pain. When exercise planed for treatment, it is necessary to have an understanding of abnormalities in the muscular system associated with painful dysfunctional joints. Two types of exercise programs, based on the muscle deficits considered to occur in neck pain, have been proposed to address cervical flexor muscle impairment. The first exercise regime consists of general strengthening and endurance excercises for the neck flexor muscles [Jordan et al., 1998; Bronfort et al., 2001]. These exercises involve high load training and they recruit all the muscle synergists that is, both the deep and superficial muscles. This program trained the cervical flexors muscles with the controlled head lift exercise and focus on training endurance and increasing the number of repetitions [Berg et al., 1994, Bronfort et al., 2001].

The second exercise regime has been designed to focus on the muscle control aspects and aims at improving control of the muscles within the neck flexor synergy (Jull et al 2004).

Specific exercise program significantly reduced the frequency of headache and neck pain and results were maintained in the long term at the 12 month follow-up.

Spinal Manipulation

The American Chiropractic Association [2007] defines spinal manipulation as a passive manual maneuver "during which the three joint complex may be carried beyond the normal voluntary physiological range of movement into the para-physiologic space without exceeding the boundaries of anatomic integrity. Most of spinal manipulation studies focus on low back pain which showed it was not superior to pharmacological interventions [Assendelft et al., 2003].

The mechanisms responsible for the effective pain relief and restoration of functional ability documented after spinal manipulation of dysfunctional cervical joints may be due to alteration in specific central corticomotor facilitatory and inhibitory neural processing and cortical motor control of upper limb muscles in a muscle-specific manner [Taylor and Murphy, 2008].

One study showed that C7-T1 spinal manipulation improved the pain pressure threshold in health individuals without a current history of neck pain in C5-C6 zygapophyseal joints [de-Las-Peñas et al., 2008]. Spinal manipulation, if not contraindicated, may be the only treatment modality of the assessed regimens that provides broad and significant long-term benefit compared with acupuncture or medications [Muller and Giles, 2005]. Data of three randomized controlled trials consisted of 329 patients with non-specific neck pain in an adult (18-70years) showed that up to 25% clinically relevant improvement in pain [Schellingerhout et al., 2008].

Nutraceuticals

The recent recommendations of American College of Rheumatology (ACR) guidelines for treating OA [2000] included dietary supplements, such as glucosamine sulfate, chondroitin sulfate, and antioxidants, as well as acupuncture and magnets as therapies under investigation.

Glucosamine

Glucosamine is an amino sugar and a prominent precursor in the biochemical synthesis of glycosylated proteins and lipids. Since glucosamine is a precursor for glycosaminoglycans, and glycosaminoglycans are a major component of joint cartilage, supplemental glucosamine may help to rebuild cartilage and treat arthritis. In the United States, glucosamine is not approved by the Food and Drug Administration for medical use in humans. It has the following pharmacological actions:

(a) Antiinflammatory [Largo et al., 2003;Chan et al., 2006]
(b) Stimulates the synthesis of proteoglycans [Bassleer et al., 1998]
(c) Reduces the catabolic activity of chondrocytes by inhibiting the synthesis of proteolytic enzymes and other substances that contribute to damage cartilage matrix [Dodge and Jimenez, 2003; Chan et al., 2005]

There have been multiple clinical trials of glucosamine as a medical therapy for osteoarthritis, but results have been conflicting. Reginster et al [2001] and Pavelka et al [2002] showed a clear benefit for glucosamine treatment while Hughes and Carr [2002] and Cibere et al [2004] did not detect any benefit of glucosamine. Some reviews and meta-analyses have evaluated the efficacy of glucosamine. Richy et al [2003] performed a meta-analysis of randomized clinical trials in 2003 and found glucosamine efficacy on VAS and Western Ontario MacMaster Questionnaire (WOMAC) pain, Lequesne index and visual analog scales (VAS) mobility and good tolerability. Recently, a review by Bruyere and Reginster [2007] about glucosamine and chondroitin sulfate for the treatment of knee and hip osteoarthritis concluded that both products act as valuable symptomatic therapies for osteoarthritis disease with some potential structure-modifying effects. OsteoArthritis Research Society International (OARSI) is recommending glucosamine as the second most effective treatment for moderate cases of osteoarthritis.In vitro, experimental study of interleukin-1 (IL-1) stimulated rat, glucosamine completely inhibited IL-6 and TNF-alpha and increased nitric oxide with no effect to annulus cells viability [Walsh et al., 2007].

Chondroitin Sulfate

It is a sulfated glycosaminoglycan composed of a chain of alternating sugars (N-acetylgalactosamine and glucuronic acid). It is usually found attached to proteins as part of a proteoglycan. Chondroitin sulfate is an important structural component of cartilage and provides much of its resistance to compression. It is approved and regulated as a symptomatic slow-acting drug for osteoarthritis in Europe and some other countries [Jordan and Arden, 2003].

Methylsulfonylmethane
It is an organosulfur compound with colorless solid. It occurs naturally in some primitive plants and is present in small amounts in many foods and beverages. Usha and Naidu [2004] found that 1500 mg per day methylsulfonylmethane (alone or in combination with glucosamine sulfate) was helpful in relieving symptoms of knee osteoarthritis. Moreover, Kim et al [2006] reported that patients, with osteoarthritis of knee, treated with methylsulfonylmethane for several weeks had significantly reduced pain and improved physical functioning, without major adverse events.

Avocado-Soybean Unsaponifiables

This preparation was superior in both pain control and functional measures in patients with osteoarthritis [Ernst, 2003].

Omega-3- fatty acids
Fish oil is rich in omega-3-fatty acids have antiinflammatory activity through their effects on prostaglandin metabolism. Several randomized controlled trials have shown clinical benefit of fish oil supplementation in rheumatoid arthritis [McCarthy and Kenny, 1992].

S-Adenosyl Methionine
It is one of the dietary supplements that gained popularity, and was recently reported to be effective in the management of depression, liver disease and arthritis. It is produced endogenously from methionine and adenosine triphosphate (ATP). It is an important methyl group donor playing an essential role in many biochemical reactions involving enzymatic transmethylation that play an important role in the biosynthesis of phospholipids that are important for the integrity of cell membranes. In *in vitro* studies using human articular chondrocytes have shown SAMe-induced increases in proteoglycan synthesis [Harmand et al., 1987] and proliferation rates in rabbits [Barcelo et al., 1987].

SAMe may reduce inflammatory mediators thus reducing pain. This was noted in other studies with the reduction of TNF-α and fibronectin RNA expression using cultured rabbit synovial cells [Gutierrez et al., 1997]. SAMe has a slower onset of action but is as effective as celecoxib in the management of symptoms of knee osteoarthritis [Najm et al., 2004]. It improves, possibly through analgesic and anti-inflammatory properties, the disease activity, pain, fatigue, morning stiffness and mood of patients with fibromyalgia [Jacobson et al., 1991].

In brief, potential mechanisms of nutraceuticals in osteoarthritis include:

(a) Increase the synthesis of glycosaminoglycan , prostaglandins and hyaluronic acid
(b) Increase synthesis of aggrecan
(c) Inhibit metalloproteinase involved in cartilage breakdown.
(d) Inhibit IL-1 induced increases aggercanases activity
(e) Inhibit nitric oxide production induced by IL-1 and TNF

Herbal Medicines

The most popular forms of complementary treatments are herbal medicines. In the United States, the annual expenditure on herbal remedies exceeds 1.5 billion dollars and grows each year by approximately 25% [Muller and Clauson, 1997]. Most of the herbal medicines have an effect on the eicosanoid metabolism, inhibiting one or both of the cyclooxygenase and lipoxygenase pathways. Ideal extract doses and treatment periods still have to be determined. In most cases, herbal treatments are based on traditional use, which is a notoriously unreliable indicator of effectiveness [Ernst, 1998]. Herbal medicines are advantageous because they do not have dangerous adverse reactions that occurred from long-term use of steroids or non steroidal anti-inflammatory drugs. The following herbs are traditionally used as analgesics:

Cayenne (Capsicum Frutescens)

The active ingredient of cayenne is capsaicin. Patients with fibromyalgia receiving the active therapy (capsaicin plasters) experienced less tenderness and significant increase in grip strength [McCarthy et al., 1994; Gagnier et al., 2007].

St John's Wort (Hypericum Perforatum)

It affects nerve and is effective for sharp, shooting nerve pains. In laboratory animals, Hypericum perforatum extract shows significant antinociceptive effect and it potentiates morphine induced antinociceptive effect [Uchida et al., 2008].

Siberian Gingseng

It resolves the fatigue associated with fibromyalgia.

Tumeric

It reduces pain and inflammation. Curcumin is the active compound in tumeric. Curcumin is effective as cortisone and phenylbutazone in decreasing inflammation. It blocks the effect of substance P on neuron besides it reduces the levels of prostaglandins, TNF-alpha and nitric oxide [Sharma et al., 2007].

Calendula officinalis (also known as marigold)

In Italian folk medicine calendula is used as an antipyretic and anti-inflammatory. It is used to revere symptoms of fibromyalgia. Recently it is studied in combination with other natural product, as direct anticytokine therapy with maximum anti-inflammatory on cell model of inflammation [Gorchakova et al., 2007].

Devil's Claw Root (Harpagophytum Procumbens)

It is a natural anti-inflammatory used to treat rheumatic disorders. The herbal preparation was reported as significantly better than placebo for pain reduction and increased the mobility in patients with osteoarthritis [Guyader, 1984; Lecomte and Costa, 1992].

Willow Bark (Salix Alba)

It contains a chemical similar to aspirin. The active ingredient is salicin which is transformed in the stomach to salicylic acid. Willow bark extracts have analgesic, antiinflammatory and antipyretic effects and therefore may be important in treatment of neck pain. There is evidence that willow bark has short term improvement in pain of spine [Gagnier et al., 2007].

Feverfew (Tanacetum parthenium) sometimes called A "Summer Daisy

It has analgesic and anti-inflammatory properties due to reducing the prostaglandins production. The active ingredient is parthenolide that inhibits the prostaglandins production but it does not inhibit cyclooxygenases [Kwok et al., 2001]. Parthenolide also specifically binds to and inhibits IκB kinase complex (IKK)β, an important proinflammatory cytokine [Collier et al.,1980; Brown et al., 1997].

Dong Quai (Radix Angelicae sinesis) also known as Chinese angalica, female ginseng It is good for fleeting muscle and joint pains. Dong quai is traditionally used in the treatment of arthritis. However, there is insufficient reliable human evidence to recommend the use of Dong quai alone or in combination with other herbs for osteoarthritis or rheumatoid arthritis.

Licorice (Glycyrrhiza glabra) root: it acts in the body like cortisone. Licorice, ginseng, bupleurum stimulate the pituitary and adrenal glands to increase natural production of cortisone [Wu, 2008].Because licorice can affect the metabolism of steroids, licorice is sometimes used to decrease inflammation.

Dandelion (Taraxacum officinale): it reduces frequency and intensity of pain and strength the connective tissue. In laboratory animals dandelion root may possess anti-inflammatory properties but there is a lack of well-conducted human studies in this area.

Ginger (Zingiber officinale) tea: it is good alternative to aspirin to relieve minor aches and pains. It has long been used in India to treat inflammation and pain. It relieves the pain of muscle spasm, rheumatoid arthritis and osteoarthritis by lowering prostaglandins level [Frondoza et al., 2004; Shen et al., 2005; Lantz et al., 2007]

Pomegrante(Punica Granatum L.)

Extracts of pomegranate fruit have been shown to possess anti-inflammatory and cartilage sparing effects *in vitro* [Ahmed et al., 2005]. It has been shown that pomegranate extract exerted a powerful influence in inhibiting the expression of inflammatory cytokines IL-1and IL-6 in adjunctive periodontal therapy [Sastravaha et al., 2005]. Shukla et al [2008] found that pomegranate extract inhibits the IL-1-induced PGE2 and NO production in rabbit chondrocytes, and also inhibits both COX-1 and COX-2 enzyme activity *ex vivo* but the effect was more pronounced on the enzyme activity of COX-2 enzyme.

Gamma-Linolenic Acid (GLA)-Containing Herbs

Blackcurrant (*Ribes nigrum*) seeds contain high levels of GLA, an essential fatty acid that exerts anti-inflammatory activity by interfering with prostaglandin metabolism [Darlington and Stone, 2001]. It suppresses the release of inflammatory mediators, perhaps by direct effect on T cell. It showed significant reduction in pain as compared with placebo in patients with rheumatoid arthritis. In one randomized controlled study, blackcurrant seed oil did not show objective signs of reduced activity of rheumatoid arthritis [Levanthal et al., 1994].

Boswellia (Boswellia Serrata)

Ayurvedic medicine is an ancient system of healing that originated in India over 4000 years ago. Ayurvedic preparation, has demonstrated anti-inflammatory activity in vitro by reducing leukotriene synthesis [Ammon et al., 1993].

Pine-bark extract: it is natural anti-inflammatory
Grape seeds extract: it is natural anti-inflammatory

Moreover, topical application of Cayenne (Capsicum) mixed with wintergreen oil can help to relieve muscle pain and the following mixture of passion flower, valerian hops tea have sedative and muscle relaxant properties. *Phytodolor* is a standardised herbal preparation of *Populus tremula*, *Fraxinus excelsior* and *Solidago virgaurea* (ratio 3:1:1) used for the treatment of musculoskeletal pain. It may have anti-inflammatory properties, and it is thought to inhibit arachidonic acid metabolism via the cyclooxygenase and lipoxygenase pathways, leading to suppression of inflammation. Significant pain relief and joint mobility was observed in rheumatoid patients received this herbal preparation [Ernst and Chrubasik, 2000; Ernst, 1999].

Certain active ingredients are extracted from herbs and plants are used as analgesics. Examples of these substances are quercetin and bromelain. *Quercetin* is a flavonol. It found in capers, lovage, apples, tea, onion espicailly red onion, red grapes, citrus fruit, tomato, leafy green vegetables and in varieties of honey. Quercetin has demonstrated significant anti-inflammatory activity because of direct inhibition of several initial processes of inflammation including inhibition of inflammatory leukotriene production. It inhibits both the synthesis and release of histamine and other allergic/inflammatory mediators. In addition, it exerts potent antioxidant and anti-tumor properties [Paliwal et al., 2005]. Experimentally, it inhibits uric acid production in a manner similar to allopurinol, as well as inhibits synthesis and release of inflammatory compounds. In animals Quercetin induces an antinociceptive effect and when combined with clonidine produces a synergistic analgesic effect [Kaur et al., 2005]. *Bromelain* is an enzyme from the stem of the pine apple, inhibits prostaglandins production and reduces the inflammation due to arthritis or sport injury [Klein and Kullich, 1999]. It is currently used for pain relief in a number of US hospitals.

VI. QUALITY OF LIFE

There is no doubt that neck pain can influence the patient's quality of life. There are several instruments for assessment the quality of life (QoL) in patients with pain.

Kovacs et al [2008] compared the psychometric characteristic of the Spanish version of the Northwick Pain Questionnaire with Neck Disability Index Questionnaire (NDI), and the Core Outcome Measure (COM) in patients with nonspecific chronic pain. The authors found that neck disability index seems to be the best instrument for measuring neck pain-related disability because the core outcome measure and Northwick pain questionnaire are worse and its use may lead to patients' evolution seeming more positive than it actually is.

Forestier et al [2007] suggested the Copenhagen Neck Functional Disability Scale (CNFDS) as a good tool for evaluating neck pain because its scores were normally distributed and were less sensitive to change than the visual analogue scale pain scores, the short-form-36 quality-of-life instrument (SF-36), and more sensitive to change than the other efficacy criteria. Individuals seeking care for neck or back pain have worse health status [assessed by health related quality of life and pain intensity] than those who do not seek care [Côté et al., 2001]. Health-related quality of life as measured by the SF-36 Short Form questionnaire is strongly affected by orofacial pain [Kohlmann, 2002]. Even controlling for gender, age, and number of pains during the past 7 days statistically significant reduction of scores in 5 out of 6 SF-36 subscales was observed in those with prevalent orofacial pain. Long term neck pain may influence the quality of life. Wallin and Raak [2008] evaluate the health related quality of life in whiplash associated disorder (WAD) patients using the SF-36 and found WAD patients are scored lower on the SF-36 in all scales when compared with healthy pain-free individuals. According to Bono et al data [2000] who used the short form Health Survey (SF-36), whiplash patients showed an impairment of cervical spine mobility, as well as a poor QoL, compared to a control group population

Rezai et al [2008] examined the association between grades of neck pain and, physical and mental components of health related –quality of life (HR-QOL) using SF-36 health survey. Their results showed that individuals with chronic neck pain with grade III-IV had significant lower physical and mental components, and the author attributed these findings to co-morbidities. Both standard physical therapy (including hot pack, ultrasound therapy and exercise program) traction therapy in addition to standard physical therapy improved significantly in pain intensity, the scores of neck disability index and physical subscales of quality of life assessed by Nottingham Health Profile in patients with nonspecific chronic pain [Borman et al., 2008].

Certain assessment of patients with neck pain may optimize the efficacy of rehabilitation program. Börsbo et al [2008] assessed 275 consecutive chronic pain patients with whiplash associated disorders using self-report questionnaires related to pain intensity in neck and shoulders, Beck Depression Inventory, Catastrophizing scale of coping strategy questionnaire, life satisfaction checklist, the SF-36 health survey and EurQOL. The authors found that the degree of depression appears to be the most important influencing factor to perceived health and quality of life in patients with whiplash-associated disorders. Haines et al [2008] assessed patient education strategies for neck pain at three advices focusing on activation, pain and stress coping skills and "traditional neck school" and found ineffective educational interventions in various disorder types and follow-up periods. EuroQol (EQ-5D) had the highest overall ability to predict return to work or not return to work irrespective of gender, neck or low back pain or duration of the problems in cohort of 1,575 men and women sick-listed more than 28 days due to back or neck problems [Hansson et al., 2006.] In a cross-sectional study was conducted on 2356 patients with neck pain, 171 of them who received worker's compensation showed significant lower SF-36 scores for Physical Functioning [Hee et al., 2002] Trigger point acupuncture therapy is more effective than aqupoints or non-trigger point acupuncture in reducing pain intensity and improving the quality of life in aged patients with chronic neck pain [Itoh et al., 2007]. Pulsed radiofrequency treatment of the cervical dorsal root ganglion may provide pain relief for limited number patients with chronic cervical radicular pain for a mean period of 9.2 months and significantly improved the quality of life in the SF-36 domain vitality at 3 months. There were no important differences in quality-adjusted life expectancy associated with standard non steroidal anti-inflammatory drugs, selective COX-2 inhibitors, exercise, mobilization, and manipulation in patients with nonspecific chronic pain [van der Velde et al., 2008]. Ma et al [2007] found that oxycondone controlled release could be an important optional drug for the management of refractory and frequent acute episodes of chronic neck pain, it improves the pain, sleep and quality of life as the most domains of SF-36 were improved. Neck pain had a significant impact on all SF-36 domains and represented the main determinant of depression in cervical dystonia. Botulinium neurotoxin type (A) therapy resulted in a significant improvement of clinical symptoms in cervical dystonia and only two of the eight SF-36 domains improved significantly in patients with cervical dystonia [Müller et al., 2002]. Botulinum neurotoxin type (A) treatment has some efficacy when administered within 1 year of the whiplash injury and improves the quality of life as evaluated by the SF-36 questionnaire but it does not reach to the significant level [Braker et al., 2008]. Cano et al (2006) found that the Subscales of the cervical dystonia impact profile (CDIP-58) were more sensitive in detecting statistical and clinical change than comparable subscales of the Medical Outcome Study Short Form-Health Survey (SF-36), Functional Disability Questionnaire (FDQ), and Toronto Western Spasmodic Torticollis Rating Scale (TWSTRS) in patients with cervical dystonia treated with botulinum toxin (A).

CONCLUSION

The above review has focused on specific targets and classes of drugs that are used in management of neck pain. In recognizing the complexity of causes of neck pain, it is important to take in consideration that the optimal pain relief may require combinations of more than one agent, more than one pharmaceutical preparation and sometimes spinal injections. With certain conditions like cephalogenic headache and fibromyalgia, combinations could include any number of multiple targets for pain mediators while with cervical dystonia, neurotoxins could resole the problem. Tolerance and dependence may occur in patients with chronic pain then alternative strategies may combat them. Traditional medicines play a role in management of neck pain and antimicrobials should be appropriately selected in treatment of spinal infections.

REFERENCES

Ackerman, LL; Follett, KA; Rosenquist, RW. Long-term outcomes during treatment of chronic pain with intrathecal clonidine or clonidine/opioid combinations. *J. Pain Symptom Manage,* 2003, 26, 668-677.

Agarwal, S; Polydefkis, M; Block, B; Haythornthwaite, J; Raja, SN. Transdermal fentanyl reduces pain and improves functional activity in neuropathic pain states. *Pain Med.,* 2007, 8, 554-562.

Ahmed, M; Bjurholm, A; Theodorsson, E; Schultzberg, M; Kreicbergs, A. Neuropeptide Y- and vasoactive intestinal polypeptide-like immunoreactivity in adjuvant arthritis: effects of capsaicin treatment. *Neuropeptides,* 1995, 29, 33-43.

Ahmed, S; Wang, N; Hafeez, BB; Cheruvu, VK; Haqqi, TM. *Punica granatum* L. extract inhibits IL-1beta-induced expression of matrix metalloproteinases by inhibiting the activation of MAP kinases and NF-kappaB in human chondrocytes *in vitro. J. Nutr.*, 2005, 135, 2096-2102.

Albright, AL; Gilmartin, R; Swift, P; Krach, LE; Ivanhoe, CB; McLaughlin, JF. Long term intrathecal baclofen therapy for severe spasticity of cerebral origin. *J. Neurosurg.*, 2003, 98, 291-295.

Aley, KO; Green, PG; Levine, JD. Opioid and adenosine peripheral antinociception are subject to tolerance and withdrawal. *J. Neurosci.*, 1995, 15, 8031-8038.

Allan, L; Richarz, U; Simpson, K; Slappendel, R. Transdermal fentanyl versus sustained release oral morphine in strong-opioid naïve patients with chronic low back pain. *Spine*, 2005, 30, 2484-2490.

Almekinders, LC; Baynes, AJ; Bracey, LW. An in vitro investigation into the effects of repetitive motion and nonsteroidal antiinflammatory medication on human tendon fibroblasts. *Am. J. Sports Med.*, 1995, 23,119-23.

Al-Nammari, SS; Lucas, JD; Lam, KS. Hematogenous methicillin-resistant Staphylococcus aureus spondylodiscitis. *Spine*, 2007, 32, 2480-2486.

Alvarez, DJ; Rockwell, PG. Trigger points: diagnosis and management. *Am. Fam. Physician*, 2002, 65, 653-660.

Amara, SG; Jonas, V; Rosenfeld, MG; Ong, ES; Evans, RM. Alternative RNA processing in calcitonin gene expression generates mRNAs encoding different polypeptide products. *Nature*, 1982, 298, 240–244.

American Chiropractic Association. Policy Statement on Spinal Manipulation. February 2003. Available at: http://www.acatoday.com/content_css.cfm?CID=1083.Accessed April 16, 2007.

Ammon, HP; Safayhi, H; Mack, T; Sabieraj, J. Mechanism of anti-inflammatory actions of curcumine and boswellic acids. *J. Ethnopharmacol.,* 1993, 38:113-119.

Andersson, HI; Ejlertsson, G; Leden, I; Rosenberg, C. Chronic pain in a geographically defined general population: studies of differences in age, gender, social class and pain localization. *Clin. J. Pain*, 1993, 9, 174-182.

Anderson, VC; Burchiel, KJ. A prospective study of long-term intrathecal morphine in the management of chronic nonmalignant pain. *Neurosurgery*, 1999, 44, 289-300.

Anderson, VC; Cooke, B; Burchiel, KJ. Intrathecal hydromorphone for chronic nonmalignant pain: A retrospective study. *Pain Med.*, 2001, 2, 287-297.

Arita, M; Bianchini, F; Aliberti, J; Sher, A; Chiang, N; Hong, S; Yang, R; Petasis, NA; Serhan, CN. Stereochemical assignment, antiinflammatory properties, and receptor for the omega-3 lipid mediator resolvin E1. *J. Exp. Med.*, 2005, 201, 713−722.

Arun, R; Kasbekar, AV; Mehdian, SM. Spontaneous kyphotic collapse followed by autostabilisation secondary to cervical osteomyelitis in an intravenous drug abuser. *Acta Orthop Belg,* 2007, 73, 807-811.

Assendelft, WJ; Morton, SC; Yu, EI; Suttorp, MJ; Shekelle, PG. Spinal manipulative therapy for low back pain: a meta-analysis of effectiveness relative to other therapies. *Ann Intern Med*, 2003, 138: 871-881

Astin, JA; Beckner, W; Soeken, K; Hochberg, MC; Berman, B. Psychological interventions for rheumatoid arthritis: a meta-analysis of randomized controlled trials. *Arthritis Rheum*, 2002, 47, 291-302.

Bablis, P; Pollard, H; Bonello, R. Neuro Emotional Technique for the treatment of trigger point sensitivity in chronic neck pain sufferers: A controlled clinical trial. *Chiropractic and Osteopathy*, 2008, 16, 4.

Baker, AS; Ojemann, RG; Swartz, MN; Richardson, EP. Spinal epidural abscess. *N. Engl. J. Med*, 1975, 293, 463-468.

Baker, R; Dreyfuss, P; Mercer, S; Bogduk, N. Cervical transforaminal injection of corticosteroids into a radicular artery: a possible mechanism for spinal cord injury. *Pain*, 2003, 103, 211-215.

Barcelo, HA; Wiemeyer, JC; Sagasta, CL; Macias, M; Barreira, JC. Effect of S-adenosylmethionine on experimental osteoarthritis in rabbits. *Am. J. Med*, 1987, 83, 55-59.

Barnes, PJ; Belvisi, MG; Rogers, DF. Modulation of neurogenic inflammation: novel approaches to inflammatory disease. *Trends Pharmacol Sci*, 1990, 11,185-189.

Barton, E; Flanagan, P; Hill, S. Spinal infection caused by ESBL-producing Klebsiella pneumoniae treated with Temocillin. *J. Infect*, 2008, 57, 347-349.

Baron, JA; Sandler, RS; Bresalier, RS; Lanas, A; Morton, DG; Riddell, R; Iverson, ER; Demets, DL. Cardiovascular events associated with rofecoxib: final analysis of the APPROVe trial. *Lancet*, 2008, 372, 1756-1764.

Barontini, F; Conti, P; Marello, G; Maurri, S. Major neurological sequelae of lumbar epidural anesthesia. Report of three cases. *Ital. J. Neurol. Sci.*, 1996, 17, 333-339.

Bassetti, M; Vitale, F; Melica, G; Righi, E; Di Biagio, A; Molfetta, L; Pipino, F; Cruciani, M; Bassetti, D. Linezolid in the treatment of Gram-positive prosthetic joint infections. *J. Antimicrob. Chemother*, 2005, 55, 387-390.

Bassleer, C Rovati, L; Franchimont, P. Stimulation of proteoglycan production by glucosamine sulfate in chondrocytes isolated from human osteoarthritic articular cartilage in vitro. *Osteoarthritis Cartilage*, 1998, 6, 427-434.

Belfrage, M; Segerdahl, M; Arnér, S; Sollevi, A. The safety and efficacy of intrathecal adenosine in patients with chronic neuropathic pain. *Anesth. Analg*, 1999, 89, 136-142.

Berbari, EF; Steckelberg, JM; Osmon, DR. Osteomyelitis. In: Mandell GL, Bennett JE, Dolin R, eds. *Mandell, Douglas, and Bennett's Principles and Practice of Infectious Diseases*. 6th ed. Oxford, England: Churchill Livingstone.; 2005:1322-1330.

Berg, HE; Berggren, G; Tesch, P. Dynamic neck strength training effect on pain and function. *Archives of Physical Medicine and Rehabilitation*, 1994, 75, 661–665.

Bernard, JM; Macaire, P. Dose-range effects of clonidine added to lidocaine for brachial plexus block. *Anesthesiology*, 1997, 87, 277-284.

Besson, M; Desmeals, J; Piguet, V. What is the place of topical analgesia in neuropathic pain. *Rev. Med.*, 2008, 4, 1500, 1502-1504.

Bihari, K. Safety, effectiveness, and duration of effect of BOTOX after switching from Dysport for blepharospasm, cervical dystonia, and hemifacial spasm dystonia, and hemifacial spasm. *Curr. Med. Res. Opin.*, 2005, 21, 433-438.

Birrell, GJ; McQueen, DS; Iggo, A; Coleman, RA; Grubb, BD. PGI2-induced activation and sensitization of articular mechanonociceptors. *Neurosci. Lett*, 1991,124, 5-8.

Black, JA; Liu, S; Tanaka, M; Cummins, TR; Waxman, SG. Changes in the expression of tetrodotoxin-sensitive sodium channels within dorsal root ganglia neurons in inflammatory pain. *Pain*, 2004, 108, 237-247.

Blossfeldt, P. Acupuncture for chronic neck pain--a cohort study in an NHS pain clinic. *Acupunct. Med.*, 2004, 22,146-151.

Bonnefont, J; Alloui, A; Chapuy, E; Clottes, E; Eschalier, A. Orally administered paracetamol does not act locally in the rat formalin test: evidence for a supraspinal, serotonin-dependent antinociceptive mechanism. *Anesthesiology*, 2003, 99, 976-981.

Bonnefont, J; Chapuy, E; Clottes, E; Alloui, A; Eschalier, A. Spinal 5-HT1A receptors differentially influence nociceptive processing according to the nature of the noxious stimulus in rats: effect of WAY-100635 on the antinociceptive activities of paracetamol, venlafaxine and 5-HT. *Pain*, 2005,114, 482-490.

Bonnetfont, J; Daulhac, L; Etienne, M; Chapuy, E; Mallet, C; Ouchuchane,L; Deval, C; Courade, J-P; ferrara, M; Eschalier, A; Clottes, E. Acetaminophen recruits spinal p42/p44 MAPKs and HH/IGF-1 receptors to produce analgesia via the serotonergic system. *Mol. Pharmacol*, 2007, 71, 407-415.

Bono, G; Antonaci, F; Ghirmai, S; D'Angelo, F; Berger, M; Nappi, G. Whiplash injuries: clinical picture and diagnostic work-up. *Clin. Exp. Rheumatol*, 2000, 18(2 Suppl 19), S23-28.

Bot, SD; Terwee, CB; van der Windt, DA; Bouter, LM; Dekker, J; de Vet, HC. Clinimetric evaluation of shoulder disability questionnaires: a systematic review of the literature. *Ann. Rheum. Dis.*, 2004, 63, 335-341.

Bot, SD; van der Waal, JM; Terwee, CB; van der Windt, DA; Schellevis, FG; Bouter, LM; Dekker, J. Incidence and prevalence of complaints of the neck and upper extremity in general practice. *Ann Rheum Dis*, 2005, 64, 118-123.

Borman, P; Keskin, D; Ekici, B; Bodur, H. The efficacy of intermittent cervical traction in patents with chronic neck pain. *Clin. Rheumatol*, 2008, 27, 1249-1253.

Börsbo, B; Peolsson, M; Gerdle, B. Catastrophizing, depression, and pain: Correlation with and influence on quality of life and health - A study of chronic whiplash-associated disorders. *J. Rehabil Me*d., 2008, 40, 562-569.

Braker, C; Yariv, S; Adler, R; Badarny, S; Eisenberg, E. The analgesic effect of botulinum-toxin A on postwhiplash neck pain. *Clin. J. Pain*, 2008, 24, 5-10.

Braun, J; McHugh, N; Singh, A; Wajdula, JS; Sato, R. Improvement in patient-reported outcomes for patients with ankylosing spondylitis treated with etanercept 50 mg once-weekly and 25 mg twice weekly. *Rheumatology* (Oxford), 2007, 46, 999-1004.

Breit, R; Nade, S .Pseudomonas osteomyelitis of the spine. Report of a case not associated with drug abuse. *Aust. N Z J. Surg.* 1987, 57, 871-873.

Brimijoin, S; Helland, L. Rapid retrograde transport of dopamine-B-hydroxylase as examined by stop-flow technique. *Brain Res.*, 1976, 102, 217-228.

Bronfort, G; Evans, R; Nelson, B; Aker, PD; Goldsmith, CH; Vernon, H. A randomized clinical trial of exercise and spinal manipulation for patients with chronic neck pain. *Spine*, 2001, 26, 788–797.

Brook, I. Two cases of diskitis attributable to anaerobic bacteria in children. *Pediatrics*, 2001,107, E26.

Brouwers, PJ; Kottink, EJ; Simon, MA; Prevo, RL. A cervical anterior spinal artery syndrome after diagnostic blockade of the right C6-nerve root. *Pain*, 2001, 91, 397-399.

Brown, AM; Edwards, CM; Davey, MR; Power, JB; Lowe, KC. Pharmacological activity of feverfew (Tanacetum parthenium [L.] Schultz-Bip.): assessment by inhibition of human polymorphonuclear leukocyte chemiluminescence in vitro. *J. Pharm Pharmacol.*, 1997, 49, 558-561.

Browning, R; Jackson, JL; O'Malley, PG. Cyclobenzaprine and back pain. A Meta analysis. *Arch. Int. Med.*, 2001, 161, 1613-1620.

Bruyere, O; Reginster, JY. Glucosamine and chondroitin sulfate as therapeutic agents for knee and hip osteoarthritis. *Drugs Aging*, 2007, 24, 573-580.

Bush, K; Hillier, S. Outcome of cervical radiculopathy treated with periradicular/epidural corticosteroid injections: a prospective study with independent clinical review. *Eur. Spine J.*, 1996, 5, 319-325.

Buskila, D; Neumann, L; Vaisberg, G; Alkalay, D; Wolfe, F. Increased rates of fibromyalgia following cervical spine injury. A controlled study of 161 cases of traumatic injury. *Arthritis Rheum.*, 1997, 40, 446-452.

Bustamante, D; Paeile, C; Willer, JC; Le Bars, D. Effects of intravenous nonsteroidal antiinflammatory drugs on a C-fiber reflex elicited by a wide range of stimulus intensities in the rat. *J Pharmacol Exp Ther*, 1996, 276, 1232-1243.

Cano, SJ; Hobart, JC; Edwards, M; Fitzpatrick, R; Bhatia, K; Thompson, AJ; Warner, TT. CDIP-58 can measure the impact of botulinum toxin treatment in cervical dystonia. *Neurology*, 2006, 67, 2230-2232.

Capasso, F; Balestrieri, B; Di Rosa, M; Persico, P; Sorrentino, L. Enhancement of carrageenin foot oedema by 1,10 -phenanthroline and evidence for the bradykinin as endogenous mediator. *Agents Actions*, 1975, 5, 359-363.

Carlsson, KC; Hoem, NO; Moberg, ER; Mathisen, LC. Analgesic effect of dextromethorphan in neuropathic pain. *Acta Anaesthesiol Scand*, 2004, 48, 328-336.

Carron H. Relieving pain with nerve blocks. *Geriatrics* 1978, 33, 49-57.

Carter, MS; Krause, JE. Structure, expression, and some regulatory mechanisms of the rat preprotachykinin gene encoding substance P, neurokinin A, neuropeptide K, and neuropeptide gamma. *J. Neurosci*, 1990, 10, 2203–2214.

Caterina, MJ; Schumacher, MA; Tominaga, M; Rosen, TA; Levine, JD; Julius D. The capsaicin receptor: a heat-activated ion channel in the pain pathway. *Nature*, 1997, 389(6653), 816-824.

Caterina, MJ; Leffler, A; Malmberg, AB; Martin, WJ; Trafton, J; Petersen-Zeitz, KR; Koltzenburg, M; Basbaum, AI; Julius, D. Impaired nociception and pain sensation in mice lacking the capsaicin receptor. *Science*, 2000, 288, 306–313.

Cazalets, JR; Bertrand, S; squalli-Houssaini, Y; Clarac, F. GABAergic control of spinal locomotor networks in the neonatal rat. *Ann. N Y Acad Sci.*, 1998, 860, 168-180.

Chan, PS; Caron, JP; Orth, MW. Short-term gene expression changes in cartilage explants stimulated with interleukin beta plus glucosamine and chondroitin sulfate. *J. Rheumatol*, 2006, 33, 1329-1340.

Chan, PS; Caron, JP; Orth, MW. Effect of glucosamine and chondroitin sulfate on regulation of gene expression of proteolytic enzymes and their inhibitors in interleukin-1-challenged bovine articular cartilage explants. *Am. J. Vet. Res.*, 2005, 66, 1870-1876.

Chandrasekharan, NV; Dai, H; Roos, KL; Evanson, NK; Tomsik, J; Elton, TS; Simmons, DL. COX-3, a cyclooxygenase-1 variant inhibited by acetaminophen and other analgesic/antipyretic drugs: cloning, structure, and expression. *Proc. Natl. Acad. Sci. USA*, 2002, 99, 13926-13931.

Chao J. Retrospective analysis of Kadian (morphine sulfate sustained-release capsules) in patients with chronic, nonmalignant pain. *Pain Med.*, 2005, 6, 262-265.

Chiang, N; Arita, M; Serhan, CN. Anti-inflammatory circuitry: lipoxin, aspirin-triggered lipoxins and their receptor ALX. *Prostaglandins Leukot Essent Fatty Acids*, 2005, 73(3-4), 163-177.

Childers, MK; Borenstein, D; Brown, RL; Gershon, S; Hale, ME; Petri, M; Wan, GJ; Laudadio, C; Harrison, DD. Low-dose cyclobenzaprine versus combination therapy with ibuprofen for acute neck or back pain with muscle spasm: a randomized trial. *Curr. Med. Res. Opin.*, 2005, 21,1485-1493.

Chou, R; Qaseem, A; Snow, V; Casey, D; Cross, JT; Shekelle, P; Owens, DK. Diagnosis and treatment of low back pain: a joint clinical practice guideline from the American College of Physicians and the American Pain Society. *Ann. Intern Med*, 2007, 147, 478-491.

Cibere, J; Kopec, JA; Thorne, A; Singer, J; Canvin, J; Robinson, DB; Pope, J; Hong, P; Grant, E; Esdaile, JM. Randomized, double-blind, placebo-controlled glucosamine discontinuation trial in knee osteoarthritis. *Arthritis Rheum*, 2004, 51, 738-745.

Civelli, O; Nothacker, HP; Reinscheid, R. Reverse physiology: discovery of the novel neuropeptide, orphanin FQ/nociceptin. *Crit. Rev. Neurobiol*, 1998, 12, 163-176.

Classen, AM; Wimbish, GH; Kupiec, TC. Stability of admixture containing morphine sulfate, bupivacaine hydrochloride, and clonidine hydrochloride in an implantable infusion system. *J. Pain Symptom Manage*, 2004, 28,603-611.

Cluzel, RA; Lopitaux, R; Sirot, J; Rampon, S. Rifampicin in the treatment of osteoarticular infections due to staphylococci. *J Antimicrob Chemother,* 1984, 13(suppl c), 23-29.

Cohen, RH; Perl, ER. Contributions of arachidonic acid derivatives and substance P to the sensitization of cutaneous nociceptors. *J. Neurophysiol.*, 1990, 64, 457-464.

Cohen, SP; Chang, AS; Larkin, T; Mao, J. The intravenous ketamine test: A predictive response tool for oral dextromethorphan treatment in neuropathic pain. *Anesth Analg*, 2004, 99, 1753-1759.

Cohen, SP; Wang, S; Chen, L; Kurihara, C; McKnight, G; Marcuson, M; Mao, J. An Intravenous Ketamine Test as a Predictive Response Tool in Opioid-Exposed Patients with Persistent Pain. *J. Pain Symptom Manage*, 2008 Sep 11

Colbert, AP; Wahbeh, H; Harling, N; Connelly, E; Schiffke, HC; Forsten, C; Gregory, WL; Markov, MS; Souder, JJ; Elmer, P; King, V. Static magnetic field therapy: A critical review of treatment parameters. *Evid Based Complement Alternat Med* 2007 Oct 4.

Collier, HO; Butt, NM; McDonald-Gibson, WJ; Saeed, SA. Extract of feverfew inhibits prostaglandin biosynthesis. *Lancet*, 1980, 2, 922-923.

Conaughty, JM; Chen, J; Martinez, OV; Chiappetta, G; Brookfield, KF; Eismont, F. Efficacy of linezolid versus vancomycin in the treatment of methicillin-resistant staphylococcus aureus discitis: a controlled animal model. *Spine*, 2006, 31, E830-E832.

Corning, JL. Spinal anesthesia and local medication of the cord. *N Y Med. J.*, 1885, 42, 483-485.

Costa, J; Espírito-Santo, C; Borges, A; Ferreira, JJ; Coelho, M; Moore, P; Sampaio, C. Botulinum toxin type B for cervical dystonia. *Cochrane Database of Systematic Reviews*, 2004, Issue 4. Art. No.: CD004315. DOI: 10.1002/14651858.CD004315.pub2.

Côté, P; Cassidy, JD; Carroll, L: The Saskatchewan Health and Back Pain Survey: The prevalence of neck pain and related disability in Saskatchewan adults. *Spine*, 1998, 23, 1689-1698.

Côté, P; Cassidy, JD; Carroll, L. The factors associated with neck pain and its related disability in the Saskatchewan population. *Spine*, 2000, 25, 1109-1117.

Côté, P; Cassidy, JD; Carroll L. The treatment of neck and low back pain: who seeks care? who goes where? *Med. Care*, 2001, 39, 956-967.

Cottle, L; Riordan, T. Infectious spondylodiscitis. *J. Infect*, 2008, 56, 401-412.

Courade, JP; Chassaing, C; Bardin, L; Alloui, A; Eschalier, A. 5-HT receptor subtypes involved in the spinal antinociceptive effect of acetaminophen in rats. *Eur. J. Pharmacol*, 2001, 432, 1-7.

Cousins, DV; Wilton, SD; Francis, BR; Gow, BL. Use of polymerase chain reaction for rapid diagnosis of tuberculosis. *J. Clin. Microbiol*, 1992, 30, 255-258.

Crawley, B; Saito, O; Malkmus, S; Fitzsimmons, B; Hua, X-Y; Yaksh, TL. Acetaminophen prevents hyperalgesia in central pain cascade. *Neurosci Lett*, 2008, 442, 50-53.

Crowley, KL. Clinical application of ketamine ointment in the treatment of sympathetically maintained pain. *Int. J. Pharm. Compound*, 1998, 2, 122-127.

Currier BL: Spinal infections. In: An HS (ed). *Principles and Techniques of Spine Surgery*. Baltimore: Williams and Wilkins; 1998; 567-603.

Dagenais, S; Yelland, MJ; Del Mar, C; Schoene, ML Prolotherapy injections for chronic low-back pain. *Cochrane Database Syst Rev*, 2007, (2), CD004059.

Dahl, JB; Kehlet, H. Non-steroidal anti-inflammatory drugs: rationale for use in severe postoperative pain. *Br. J. Anaesth*, 1991, 66, 703-712.

Danner, RL; Hartman, BJ. Update on spinal epidural abscess: 35 cases and review of the literature. *Rev. Infect Dis.*, 1987, 9, 265-274.

Darland, T; Heinriche,r MM; Grandy, DK. Orphanin FQ/nociceptin: a role in pain and analgesia, but so much more. *Trends Neurosci.*, 1998, 21, 215-221.

Darlington, LG; Stone, TW. Antioxidants and fatty acids in the amelioration of rheumatoid arthritis and related disorders. *Br. J. Nutr.*, 2001, 85, 251-269.

De Kock, M; Gautier, P; Pavlopoulou, A; Jonniaux, M; Lavand'homme, P. Epidural clonidine or bupivacaine as the sole analgesic agent during and after abdominal surgery: a comparative study. *Anesthesiology*, 1999, 90, 1354-1362. Erratum in: *Anesthesiology*, 1999, 91, 602.

De Felipe, C; Herrero, JF; O'Brien, JA; Palmer, JA; Doyle, CA; Smith, AJ; Laird, JM; Belmonte, C; Cervero, F; Hunt, SP. Altered nociception, analgesia and aggression in mice lacking the receptor for substance P. *Nature*, 1998, 392, 394-397.

de Goeij, S; Nisolle, JF; Glupczynski, Y; Delgrange, E; Delaere, B. Vertebral osteomyelitis with spinal epidural abscess in two patients with Bacteroides fragilis bacteraemia. *Acta Clin. Belg*, 2008, 63, 193-196.

de Las Peñas, CF; Alonso-Blanco, C; Miangolarra, JC. Myofascial trigger points in subjects presenting with mechanical neck pain: A blinded, controlled study. *Man. Ther*, 2007, 12, 29-33.

de Las Peñas, CF; Alonso-Blanco, C; Cleland, JA; Rodríguez-Blanco, C; Alburquerque-Sendín, F. Changes in pressure pain thresholds over C5-C6 zygapophyseal joint after a cervicothoracic junction manipulation in healthy subjects. *J. Manipulative Physiol. Ther*, 2008, 31, 332-337.

Dellemijn, PL; Vanneste, JA. Randomised double-blind active-placebo-controlled crossover trial of intravenous fentanyl in neuropathic pain. *Lancet*, 1997, 349(9054), 753-758.

Denti, M; Randelli, P; Bigoni, M; Vitale, G; Marino, MR; Fraschini, N. Pre- and postoperative intra-articular analgesia for arthroscopic surgery of the knee and arthroscopy-assisted anterior cruciate ligament reconstruction. A double-blind randomized, prospective study. *Knee Surg Sports Traumatol Arthrosc,* 1997, 5, 206-212.

Deutsch, DG; Chin, SA. Enzymatic synthesis and degradation of anandamide, a cannabinoid receptor agonist. *Biochem Pharmacol,* 1993, 46, 791-796.

Dickenson AH. Enkephalins. A new approach to pain relief? *Nature,* 1986, 320(6064), 681-682.

Dickenson, AH. Spinal cord pharmacology of pain. *Br. J. Anaesth,* 1995, 75,193-200.

Dickenson, AH; Sullivan, AF; Stanfa, LC; McQuay, HJ. Dextromethorphan and levorphanol on dorsal horn nociceptive neurons in the rat. *Neuropharmacology,* 1991, 30, 1303–1308.

Dimar, JR; Carreon, LY; Glassman, SD; Campbell, MJ; Hartman, MJ; Johnson, JR. Treatment of pyogenic vertebral osteomyelitis with anterior debridement and fusion followed by delayed posterior spinal fusion. *Spine,* 2004, 29, 326-332.

DiMarzo, V; Bisogno, T; DePetrocellis, L. Anandamide: some like it hot. *Trends Pharmacol Sci.,* 2001, 22, 346-349.

Dodge, GR Jimenez, SA. Glucosamine sulfate modulates the levels of aggrecan and matrix metalloproteinase-3 synthesized by cultured human osteoarthritis articular chondrocytes. *Osteoarthritis Cart,* 2003, 11, 424-432.

Donnerer, J; Schuligoi, R; Stein, C. Increased content and transport of substance P and calcitonin gene-related peptide in sensory nerves innervating inflamed tissue: evidence for a regulatory function of nerve growth factor in vivo. *Neuroscience,* 1992, 49, 693–698.

Dornan, WA; Vink, KL; Malen, P; Short, K; Struthers, W; Barrett, C. Site-specific effects of intracerebral injections of three neurokinins (neurokinin A, neurokinin K, and neurokinin gamma) on the expression of male rat sexual behavior. Physiol Behav, 1993, 54, 249–258.

Dray, A. Inflammatory mediators of pain. *Br. J. Anaesth,* 1995, 75, 125-131.

Dray, A. Kinins and their receptors in hyperalgesia. *Can J Pharmacol,* 1997, 75, 704-712.

Dray, A; Rang, H. The how and why of chronic pain states and the what of new analgesia therapies. *Trends Neurosci.,* 1998, 2, 315-317.

Dressler, D; Hallett, M. Immunological aspects of Botox, Dyport and Mybloc/Neurobloc. *Eur J. Neurol.,* 2006, 13 suppl 1, 11-15.

Dualé, C; Daveau, J; Cardot, JM; Boyer-Grand, A; Schoeffler,P; Dubray, C. Cutaneous amitriptyline in human volunteers: differential effects on the components of sensory information. *Anesthesiology,* 2008,108, 714-721.

Duggan, AW; Hope, PJ; Jarrott, B; Schaible, HG; Fleet-Wood,SM. Release, spread and persistenceof immunoreactive neurokininA in the dorsal hornof the cat following noxious cutaneous stimulation. Studies with antibody microprobes. *Neuroscience,* 1990, 35, 195-202.

Dykstra, DD; Mendez, A; Chaauis, D; Baxter, T; Deslauriers, L; Stuckey, M. Treatment of cervical dystonia and focal hand dystonia by high cervical continuously infused intrathecal baclofen; a report of 2 cases. *Arch. Phys. Med. Rehabil.,* 2005, 86, 830-833.

Eaton, M J; Karmally, S; Martinez, MA; Plunkett, JA; Lopez, T; Cejas, PJ. *J. Periphery Nerv Syst.,* 1999, 4, 245–257.

Edvinsson, L. New therapeutic target in primary headaches – blocking the CGRP receptor. *Expert Opin. Ther Targets*, 2003, 7, 377–383.

Eisenach, JC. Muscarinic-mediated analgesia. *Life Sci*, 1999, 64, 549-554.

Eismont, FJ; Bohlman, HH; Soni, PL; Goldberg, VM; Freehafer AA. Pyogenic and fungal vertebral osteomyelitis with paralysis. *J. Bone Joint Surg Am*, 1983, 65,19-29.

Ellrich, J; Makowska, A. Nerve growth factor and ATP excite different neck muscle nociceptors in anaesthetized mice. *Cephalalgia*, 2007, 27, 1226-1235.

Endress, C; Guyot, DR; Fata, J; Salciccioli, G. Cervical osteomyelitis due to i.v. heroin use: radiologic findings in 14 patients. *Am. J. Roentgenol.*, 1990, 155, 333-335.

England, S; Bevan, S; Docherty, RJ. PGE2 modulates the tetrodotoxin-resistant sodium current in neonatal rat dorsal root ganglion neurones via the cyclic AMP-protein kinase A cascade. *J. Physiol.*, 1996, 495(Pt 2), 429-40.

Ernst, E; Chrubasik, S. Phyto-anti-inflammatories: a systematic review of randomized, placebo-controlled, double blind trials. *Rheum. Dis. Clin. North Am.*, 2000, 1, 13-27.

Ernst, E. The efficacy of Phytodolor for the treatment of musculoskeletal pain -- a systematic review of randomized clinical trials. *Nat. Med. J.*, 1999, 2, 14-17.

Ernst, E. Usage of complementary therapies in rheumatology. A systematic review. *Clin Rheumatol*, 1998, 17, 301-305.

Ernst, E; Pittler, MH; Stevinson, C; White, AR. *The Desktop Guide to Complementary and Alternative Medicine*. Edinburgh: Mosby; 2001.

Ernst, E. Avacodo-soybean unsaponifiables (ASU) for osteoarthritis -- a systematic review. *Clin. Rheumatol.*, 2003, 22, 285-288.

Fass, RJ. Treatment of osteomyelitis and septic arthritis with cefazolin. *Antimicrob Agents Chemother*, 1978, 13, 405-411.

Fejer, R; Kyvik, KO; Hartvigsen, J: The prevalence of neck pain in the world population: a systematic critical review of the literature. *Eur Spine J*, 2006, 15, 834-848.

Ferrante , FM; Bearn, L; Rothrock, R; King, L. Evidence against trigger point injection technique for the treatment of cervicothoracic myofacial pain with with botulinium toxin type A. *Anesthsiology*, 2005, 103, 377-383.

Fischer, AA. Pressure threshold meter: its use for quantification of tender spots. *Arch. Phys. Med Rehabil*, 1986, 67, 836-838.

Fitzgerald, M; Woolf, CJ. The time course and specificity of the changes in the behavioural and dorsal horn cell responses to noxious stimuli following peripheral nerve capsaicin treatment in the rat. *Neuroscience*, 1982, 7, 2051–2056.

Forestier, R; Françon, A; Saint, Arroman, F; Bertolino, C. French version of the Copenhagen neck functional disability scale. *Joint Bone Spine*, 2007, 74, 155-159.

França, DL; Senna-Fernandes, V; Cortez, CM; Jackson, MN; Bernardo-Filho, M; Guimarães, MA. Tension neck syndrome treated by acupuncture combined with physiotherapy: A comparative clinical trial (pilot study). *Complement Ther Med*, 2008, 16, 268-277.

Frank, C; Amiel, D; Woo, SL-Y; Akeson, W. Normal ligament properties and ligament healing. *Clin. Ortho. Res* 1985, 196, 15-25.

Freund, BJ; Schwartz, M. Treatment of whiplash associated neck pain [corrected] with botulinum toxin-A: a pilot study. *J. Rheumatol.*, 2000, 27, 481-484.

Frondoza, CG; Sohrabi, A; Polotsky, A; Phan, PV; Hungerford, DS; Lindmark, L. An in vitro screening assay for inhibitors of proinflammatory mediators in herbal extracts using human synoviocyte cultures. *In Vitro Cell Dev. Biol. Anim*, 2004, 40, 95-101.

Fuentes, JA; Ruiz-Gayo, M; Manzanares, J; Vela, G; Reche, I; Corchero, J. Cannabinoids as potential new analgesics. *Life Sci*, 1999, 65, 675-685.

Ga, H; Choi, JH; Park, CH; Yoon, HJ. Acupuncture needling versus lidocaine injection of trigger points in myofascial pain syndrome in elderly patients--a randomised trial. *Acupunct Med*, 2007, 25, 130-136.

Gagnier, JJ; Van Tulder, MW; Berman, B; Bombardier, C. Herbal medicine for low back pain: a Cochrane review. *Spine*, 2007, 32, 82-92.

Gaillard JM. Comparison of two muscle relaxant drugs on human sleep: diazepam and parachlorophenylgaba. *Acta Psychiatr Belg*, 1977, 77, 410-425.

Gaumann, DM; Brunet, BC; Jirounek, P. Hyperpolarization after potentials in C-fibers and local anesthetic effects of clonidine and lidocaine. *Pharmacology*, 1994, 48, 21-29.

Gaumann, D; Forster, A; Griessen, M; Habre, W; Poinsot, O; Della Santa, D. Comparison between clonidine and epinephrine admixture to lidocaine in brachial plexus block. *Anesth Analg*, 1992, 75, 69-74.

Gazerani, P; Staahl, C; Drewes, AM; Arendt-Nielsen, L. The effects of Botulinum Toxin type A on capsaicin-evoked pain, flare, and secondary hyperalgesia in an experimental human model of trigeminal sensitization. *Pain*, 2006, 122, 315-325.

Genevay, S; Stingelin, S. Efficacy of etanercept in the treatment of acute, severe sciatica : a pilot study. *Annals of the Rheumatic Diseases*, 2004, 63, 1120-1123.

Gerwin, RD. Myofascial and visceral pain syndromes: visceral somatic pain representations. *J Musculoskeletal Pain*, 2002, 10, 165-175.

Gilron, I; Booher, SL; Rowan, MS; Smoller, MS; Max, MB. A randomized, controlled trial of high-dose dextromethorphan in facial neuralgias. *Neurology*, 2000, 55, 964-971.

Gorchakova, TV; Suprun, IV; Sobenin, IA; Orekhov, AN. Use of natural products in anticytokine therapy. *Bull. Exp. Biol. Med.*, 2007, 143, 316-319.

Gottrup, H; Bach, FW; Arendt-Nielsen, L; Jensen, TS. Peripheral lidocaine but not ketamine inhibits capsaicin-induced hyperalgesia in humans. *Br. J. Anaesth*, 2000, 85, 520-528.

Gottrup, H; Bach, FW; Jensen, TS. Differential effects of peripheral ketamine and lidocaine on skin flux and hyperalgesia induced by intradermal capsaicin in humans. *Clin. Physiol Funct Imaging*, 2004, 24, 103-108.

Graziani, AL; Lawson, LA; Gibson, GA; Steinberg, MA; MacGregor, RR. Vancomycin concentrations in infected and noninfected human bone. *Antimicrob Agents Chemother*, 1988, 32, 1320-1322.

Guo, YQ; Chen, LY; Fu, WB; Xu, MZ; Ou, XM. Clinically randomized controlled study on abdominal acupuncture for treatment of cervical spondylosis. *Zhongguo Zhen Jiu*, 2007, 27, 652-656.

Gureje, O; Akinpelu, AO; Uwakwe, R; Udofia, O; Wakil, A. Comorbidity and impact of chronic spinal pain in Nigeria. *Spine*, 2007, 32, E495-500.

Gutierrez, S; Palacios, I; Sanchez-Pernaute, O; Hernández, P; Moreno, J; Egido, J; Herrero-Beaumont, G. SAMe restores the changes in the proliferation and in the synthesis of fibronectin and proteoglycans induced by tumour necrosis factor alpha on cultured rabbit synovial cells. *Br. J. Rheumatol*, 1997, 36, 27-31.

Guyader, M. Les palantes antirheumatismales. Etudes historique et pharmalogique, et etude clinique du nebulisat d'Harpagophytum procumbens DC chez 50 patients arthroques sulvis en service hospitalier. Paris: Universite Pierre et Marie Curie; 1984. (Dissertation).

Hackett G. Low back pain. *Indust Med Surg*, 1959, 28, 416-419.

Hackett, G; Hemwall, G; Montgomery, G. *Ligament and tendon relaxation treated by prolotherapy*. 5th ed. Gustav A. Hemwall; Oak Park, IL; 1992.

Hadjipavlou, AG; Mader, JT; Necessary, JT; Muffoletto, AJ. Hematogenous pyogenic spinal infections and their surgical management. *Spine*, 2000, 25, 1668-1679.

Haines, T; Gross, A; Goldsmith, CH; Perry, L. Patient education for neck pain with or without radiculopathy. *Cochrane Database Syst Rev*, 2008, (4):CD005106.

Hansen, C; Gilron, I; Hong, M. The effect of intrathecal gabapentinon spinal morphine tolerance in rat tail-flickand paw pressure test. *Anesth analg*, 2004, 99,1180-1184.

Hansson, E; Hansson, T; Jonsson, R. Predictors for work ability and disability in men and women with low-back or neck problems. *Eur. Spine J.*, 2006, 15, 780-793.

Hanten, WP; Olsen, SL; Butts, NL; Nowicki, AL. Effectiveness of a home program of ischaemic pressure followed by sustained stretch for treatment of myofascial trigger points. *Phys. Ther*, 2000, 80, 997-1003.

Harmand, MF; Vilamitjana, J; Maloche, E; Duphil, R; Ducassou, D: Effects of S-adenosylmethionine on human articular chondrocyte differentiation. An *in vitro* study. *Am. J. Med.*, 1987, 83, 48-54.

Hashimoto, A; Hayashi, I; Murakami, Y; Sato, Y; Kitasato, H; Matsushita, R; Iizuka, N; Urabe, K; Itoman, M; Hirohata, S; Endo, H. Antiinflammatory mediator lipoxin A4 and its receptor in synovitis of patients with rheumatoid arthritis. *J. Rheumatol*, 2007, 34, 2144-2153.

Hassenbusch, SJ; Stanton-Hicks, M; Covington, EC; Walsh, JG; Guthrey, DS. Long term intraspinal infusions of opioids in the treatment of neuropathic pain. *J. Pain Symptom Manage*, 1995, 10, 527- 543.

Hauser, RA. Punishing the pain. Treating chronic pain with prolotherapy. *Rehab Manag* 1999, 12, 26-28, 30.

Hauser, RA; Hauser, MA. Dextrose prolotherapy for unresolved neck pain. *Practical Pain Management*, 2007, Oct, 56-69.

Hee, HTIII; Whitecloud, TS; Myers, L; Roesch, W; Ricciardi, JE. Do worker's compensation patients with neck pain have lower SF-36 scores? *Eur Spine J*, 2002, 11, 375-381.

Heppelmann B, Pawlak M. Sensitisation of articular afferents in normal and inflamed knee joints by substance P in the rat. *Neurosci. Lett*, 1997, 223, 97-100.

Heyneman ,CA; Lawless-Liday, C; Wall, GC. Oral versus topical NSAIDs in rheumatic diseases: a comparison. *Drugs* 2000, 60, 555-574.

Hildebrand, KR; Elsberry, DD; Deer, TR. Stability, compatibility, and safety of intrathecal bupivacaine administered chronically via an implantable delivery system. *Clin. J. Pain*, 2001, 17, 239-244.

Hinman, M: The therapeutic use of magnets: a review of recent research. *Phys. Ther. Rev.* 2002, 7, 33-43.

Hirota, K; Lambert, DG. Ketamine: its mechanism(s) of action and unusual clinical uses. *Br. J. Anaesth*, 1996, 77, 441–444.

Ho, KY; Huh, BK; White, WD; Yeh, CC; Miller, EJ. .Topical amitriptyline versus lidocaine in the treatment of neuropathic pain. *Clin. J. Pain*, 2008, 24, 51-55.

Hodges, SD; Castleberg, RL; Miller, T; Ward, R; Thorburg, C. Cervical epidural steroid injection with intrinsic spinal cord damage: two case reports. *Spine*, 1998, 23, 2137-2142.

Hogan, KA; Manning, EL; Glaser, JA. Progressive cervical kyphosis associated with botulinum toxin injection. *South Med. J.*, 2006, 99, 888-891.

Hökfelt, T; Wiesenfeld-Hallin, Z; Villar, M; Melander, T. Increase of galanin-like immunoreactivity in rat dorsal root ganglion cells after peripheral axotomy. *Neurosci. Lett*, 1987, 83, 217-220.

Hökfelt, T; Zhang, X; Wiesenfeld-Hallin, Z. Messenger plasticity in primary sensory neurons following axotomy and its functional implications. *Trends Neurosci*, 1994, 17, 22-30.

Holthusen, H; Arndt, JO. Nitric oxide evokes pain in humans on intracutaneous injection. *Neurosci Lett*, 1994, 165(1-2), 71-74.

Hong, C-Z; Chen, Y-C; Pon, CH; Yu J. Immediate effects of various physical medicine modalities on pain threshold of the active myofascial trigger points. *J. Musculoskel Pain*, 1993, 1, 37-52.

Hooper, RA; Frizzell, JB; Faris, P. Case series on chronic whiplash related neck pain treated with intraarticular zygapophysial joint regeneration injection therapy. *Pain Physician*, 2007, 10, 313-318.

Hughes, R; Carr, A. A randomized, double-blind, placebo-controlled trial of glucosamine sulphate as an analgesic in osteoarthritis of the knee. *Rheumatology* (Oxford), 2002, 41, 279-284.

Hsieh, C-YJ; Hong, C-Z. Effect of chiropractic manipulation on the pain threshold of myofascial trigger point. *Proceedings of the 1990 International Conference of Spinal Manipulation: Los Angeles College of Chiropractic; Los Angeles* 1990.

Hsueh, TC; Cheng, PT; Kuan, TS; Hong, CZ. The immediate effectiveness of electrical nerve stimulation and electrical muscle stimulation on myofascial trigger points. *Am J Phys Med. Rehabil*, 1997, 76, 471- 476.

Hylden, JKL; Wilcox, GL. Intrathecal substance P elicits a caudally-directed biting and scrathing behavior in mice. *Brain Res.*, 1981, 217, 212-215.

Inan, N; Yilmaz, G; Surer, H; Coskun, O; Ucler, S; Cavdar, L; Inan, LE . Is there a role for nitric oxide activity in cervicogenic headache? *Funct Neurol*, 2007, 22, 155-157.

Incavo, SJ; Ronchetti, PJ; Choi, JH; Wu, H; Kinzig, M; Sörgel, F. Penetration of piperacillin-tazobactam into cancellous and cortical bone tissues. *Antimicrob Agents Chemother*, 1994, 38, 905-907.

Inoue, Y; Koga, K; Sata, T; Shigematusa, A. Effect of fentanyl on emergence characteristics from anesthesia in adult cervical spine surgery: a comparison of fentanyl-based and sevoflurane-based anesthesia. *J. Anesth*, 2005, 19, 12-16.

Itoh, K; Katsumi, Y; Hirota, S; Kitakoji, H. Randomised trial of trigger point acupuncture compared with other acupuncture for treatment of chronic neck pain. *Complement Ther. Med.*, 2007, 15, 172-179.

Iversen, L. Substance P equals pain substance? *Nature* 1998, 392, 334-335.

Iversen, LL. Substance P. *Brit. Med. Bull*, 1982, 38, 277-282.

Iversen, LL; Chapman, V. Cannabinoids: a real prospect for pain relief? *Current Opin. Pharmacol*, 2002, 2, 50-55.

Jacobson, S; Danneskield-Samsone, B; Anderson, RB. Oral S-adenosyl methionine in primary fibromyalgia, double-blind clinical evaluation. *Scand. J. Rheumatol.*, 1991, 20, 294-302.

Janda, V. Muscles and motor control in cervicogenic disorders: assessment and management. In: Grant R, editor. *Physical therapy ofthe cervical and thoracic spine*. New York: Churchill Livingstone; 1994;195–216.

Jeal, W; Benfield, P. Transdermal fentanyl. A review of its pharmacological properties and therapeutic efficacy in pain control. *Drugs*, 1997, 53,109-138.

Jensen, AG; Espersen, F; Skinhøj, P; Rosdahl, VT; Frimodt-Møller, N. Increasing frequency of vertebral osteomyelitis following Staphylococcus aureus bacteraemia in Denmark 1980-1990. *J. Infect.*, 1997, 34,113-118.

Jessell, TM; Iversen, LL. Opiate analgesics inhibit substance P release from rat trigeminal nucleus. *Nature*, 1977, 268(5620), 549-551.

Jhaveri, MD; Elmes, SJ; Richardson, D; Barrett, DA; Kendall, DA; Mason, R; Chapman, V. Evidence for a novel functional role of cannabinoid CB receptors in the thalamus of neuropathic rats. *Eur. J. Neurosci.*, 2008, 27, 1722-1730.

John Hurlebert R. Methylprednisolone for acute spinal cord injury: an inappropriate standard of care. *J. Neurosurg. (Spine* 1), 2000, 93, 1-7.

Jordan, A; Bendix, T; Nielsen, H; Hansen, F; Host, D; Winkel, A. Intensive training, physiotherapy, or manipulation for patients with chronic neck pain. *Spine*, 1998, 23, 311–319.

Jordan, KM; Arden, NK. EULAR Recommendations 2003: an evidence based approach to the management of knee osteoarthritis: Report of a Task Force of the Standing Committee for International Clinical Studies Including Therapeutic Trials (ESCISIT). *Ann. Rheum Dis.*, 2003, 62, 1145–1155.

Jull, G; Falla, D; Treleaven, J; Sterling, M;O'Leary, S. A therapeutic exercise approach for cervical disorders. In: *Grieve's modern manual therapy: the vertebral column*, 2004.

Kabat-Zinn, J; Lipworth, I; Burney, R. Four- year follow-up of a meditation-based program for the self regulation of chronic pain: treatment outcomes and compliance. *Clin. J. Pain*, 1987, 2, 159-173.

Kabat-Zinn, J; Lipworth, I; Burney, R. The clinical use of mindfulness meditation for the self-regulation of chronic pain. *J. Behav. Med*, 1985, 8, 163-190.

Kang, JD; Georgescu, HI; McIntyre-Larkin, L; Stefanovic-Racic, M; Evans, CH. Herniated cervical intervertebral discs spontaneously produce matrix metalloproteinases, nitric oxide, interleukin-6, and prostaglandin E2. *Spine*, 1995, 20, 2373-2378.

Kangrga, I; Randić, M. Outflow of endogenous aspartate and glutamate from the rat spinal dorsal horn in vitro by activation of low- and high-threshold primary afferent fibers. Modulation by mu-opioids. *Brain Res*, 1991, 553, 347-352.

Kaur, R; Singh, D; Chopra, K. Participation of alpha2 receptors in the antinociceptive activity of quercetin. *J Med Food*, 2005, 8, 529-532.

Kim, K-H; Choi, S-H; Kim, T-K; Shin, SW. Cervical Facet Joint Injections in the Neck and Shoulder Pain. *J. Korean Med Sci*, 2005, 20, 659-662.

Kim, LS; Axelrod, LJ; Howard, P; Buratovich, N; Waters, RF. Efficacy of methylsulfonylmethane (MSM) in osteoarthritis pain of the knee: a pilot clinical trial. *Osteoarthritis Cartilage*, 2006, 14, 286–294.

Kim, SM; Kim, J; Kim, E; Hwang, SJ; Shin, HK; Lee, SE. Local application of capsaicin alleviates . *Neurosci. Lett*, 2008 , 433, 199-204.

Kissin, I; Bright,CA; Bradley, EL. Selective and Long-Lasting Neural Blockade with Resiniferatoxin Prevents Inflammatory Pain Hypersensitivity. Anesth. Analg. 2002, 94, 1253-1258.

Kissin, I. Vanilloid-induced conduction analgesia: selective, dose dependent, long lasting, with a low level of potential neurotoxicity. *Anesth Analg* 2008,107, 271-281.

Kitahata, LM. Pain pathways and transmission. *Yale J. Biol. Med.* 1993, 66, 437-442.

Klein, G; Kullich, W. Reducing pain by oral enzyme therapy in rheumatic diseases. *Wien Med Wochenschr*, 1999, 149, 577-580.

Klein AW. Complications and adverse reactions with the use of botulinum toxin. *Dis. Mon.*, 2002, 48, 336-356.

Kohane, DS; Kuang, Y; Lu, NT; Langer, R; Strichartz, GR; Berde CB. Vanilloid receptor agonists potentiate the *in vivo* local anesthetic activity of percutaneously injected site 1 sodium channel blockers. *Anesthesiology*, 1999; 90: 524–34.

Kohlmann T. Epidemiology of orofacial pain. *Schmerz*, 2002, 16, 339-345.

Kolesnikov, Y; Pasternak, GW. Topical opioids in mice: analgesia and reversal of tolerance by a topical N-methyl-D-aspartate antagonist. *J. Pharmacol Exp. Ther*, 1999, 290, 247-252.

Kolstad, F; Leivseth, G; Nygaard, O. Transforaminal steroid injections in the treatment of cervical radiculopathy. A prospective outcome study. *Acta Neurochi. (Wein)*, 2005, 147, 1065-1070.

Kosuge, S; Inagaki, Y; Okumura, H. Studies on the pungent principles of red pepper. Part VIII on the chemical contributions of the pungent principles. Nippon Nogei Kagaka (*J. Agri. Chem. Soc.*) 1961, 35, 923-927.

Kosuge, S; Inagaki, Y. Studies on the pungent principles of red pepper. Part XI. Determination and contents of the two pungent principles. Nippon Nogei Kagaka (*J. Agri. Chem. Soc.*) 1962, 36, 251.

Kovacs, FM; Bago, J; Royuela, A; Seco, J; Gimenez, S. Research Network SB Psychometric characteristics of the Spanish version of instruments to measure neck pain disability. *BMC Musculoskelet Disord*, 2008, 9, 42.

Krames, ES. Intrathecal infusional therapies for intractable pain: Patient management guidelines. *J. Pain Symptom Manage*, 1993, 8, 36-46.

Kuraishi, Y; Kawamura, M; Yamaguchi, T; Houtani, T; Kawabata, S; Futaki, S; Fujii, N; Satoh, M. Intrathecal injections of galanin and its antiserum affect nociceptive response of rat to mechanical, but not thermal, stimuli. *Pain*, 1991, 44, 321-324.

Kutscha-Lissberg, F; Hebler, U; Muhr, G; Köller, M. Linezolid penetration into bone and joint tissues infected with methicillin-resistant staphylococci. *Antimicrob Agents Chemother*, 2003, 47, 3964-3966.

Kwok, BH; Koh, B; Ndubuisi, MI; Elofsson, M; Crews, CM. The anti-inflammatory natural product parthenolide from the medicinal herb Feverfew directly binds to and inhibits IkappaB kinase. *Chem. Biol.,* 2001, 8, 759-766.

Laird, JM; Carter, AJ; Grauert, M; Cervero F. Analgesic activity of a novel use-dependent sodium channel blocker, crobenetine, in mono-arthritic rats. *Br. J. Pharmacol*, 2001, 134, 1742-1748.

Lantz, RC; Chen, GJ; Sarihan, M; Sólyom, AM; Jolad, SD; Timmermann, BN. The effect of extracts from ginger rhizome on inflammatory mediator production. *Phytomedicine,* 2007, 14, 123-128.

Largo, R; Alvarez-Soria, MA; Díez-Ortego, I; Calvo, E; Sánchez-Pernaute, O; Egido, J; Herrero-Beaumont, G. Glucosamine inhibits IL-1beta-induced NFkappaB activation in human osteoarthritic chondrocytes. *Osteoarthritis Cartilage*, 2003, 11, 290-298.

Lascelles, BD; Gaynor, JS; Smith, ES; Roe, SC; Marcellin-Little, DJ; Davidson, G; Boland, E; Carr, J. Amantadine in a multimodal analgesic regimen for alleviation of refractory osteoarthritis pain in dogs. *J. Vet. Intern Med.*, 2008, 22, 53-59.

Lautenschlager J. Present state of medication therapy in fibromyalgia syndrome. *Scand. J. Rheumatol (Suppl)*, 2000, 113, 32-36.

Leadbetter,W. Soft tissue athletic injuries. In: Fu FH, (Ed): *Sports Injuries: Mechanisms, Prevention, Treatment.* Baltimore: Williams and Wilkins; 1994; 736-737.

LeBars, D; Dickenson, AH; Besson, JM. Diffuse noxious inhibitory controls. Part I: effects on dorsal horn convergent neurones in the rat; Part II: lack of effect on nonconvergent neurones, supraspinal involvement and theoretical implications. *Pain*, 1979, 6, 283-327.

Lecomte, A; Costa, JP. Harpagophytum dans l'arthrose Etudes en double insu contre placebo. *Le Magazine* 1992, 15, 27-30.

Lee, HM; Weinstein, JN; Meller, ST; Hayshi, N; Spratt, K; Gebhart, GF. The role of steroids and their effects on phospholipase A2: an animal model of radiculopathy. *Spine*, 1998, 23, 1191-1196.

Lee YW, Yaksh, TL. Pharmacology of the spinal adenosine receptor which mediates the antiallodynic action of intrathecal adenosine agonists. *J. Pharmacol Exp. Ther*, 1996, 277, 1642–1648.

Lembeck, F; Folkers, K; Donnerer, J. Analgesic effect of antagonists of substance P. *Biochem Biophys. Res. Commun*, 1981, 103, 1318-1321.

Leslie, TA; Emson, PC; Dowd, PM; Woolf, CJ. Nerve-growth factor contributes to the upregulation of GAP-43 and preprotachykinin A mRNA in primary sensory neurons following peripheral inflammation. *Neuroscience*, 1995, 67, 753–761.

Levanthal, LJ; Boyce, EG; Zurier, RB. Treatment of rheumatoid arthritis with black current seed oil. *Br. J. Rheumatol*, 1994, 33, 847-852.

Levine, JD; Fields, HL; Basbaum, AI. Peptides and the primary afferent nociceptor. *J. Neurosci.*, 1993, 13, 2273-2286.

Levine, JD; Taiwo, YO. Involvement of the mu-opiate receptor in peripheral analgesia. *Neuroscience*, 1989, 32, 571-575.

Lew, DP; Waldvogel, FA. Osteomyelitis. *N. Engl J. Med.*, 1997, 336, 999-1007.

Lin, EL; Lieu, V; Halevi, L; Shamie, AN; Wang, JC. Cervical epidural steroid injections for symptomatic disc herniations. *J. Spinal Disord Tech.*, 2006, 19, 183-186.

Lind, G; Schechtmann, G; Winter, J; Linderoth, B. Drug-enhanced spinal stimulation for pain: a new strategy. *Acta Neurochir Suppl*, 2007, 97(Pt 1), 57-63.

Liu, HX; Hökfelt, T. The participation of galanin in pain processing at the spinal level. *Trends Pharmacol Sci.*, 2002, 23, 468-474.

Liu, H; Hökfelt, T. Effect of intrathecal galanin and its putative antagonist M35 on pain behavior in a neuropathic pain model. *Brain Res*, 2000, 886(1-2), 67-72.

Lott-Duarte, AH; Dourado, L; Tostes, M; Nascimento-Carvalho, CM. Extensive spondylodiscitis with epidural abscess causing fever and lower limbs pain in a child with sickle cell disease. *J Pediatr Hematol Oncol*, 2008, 30, 70-72.

Loubser, PG; Akman, NM. Effects of intrathecal baclofen on chronic spinal cord injury pain. *J. Pain Symptom Manage*, 1996, 12, 241-247.

Lovering, AM; Walsh, TR; Bannister, GC; MacGowan, AP. The penetration of ceftriaxone and cefamandole into bone, fat and haematoma and relevance of serum protein binding to their penetration into bone. *J. Antimicrob. Chemother*, 2001, 47, 483-486.

Lovering, AM; Zhang, J; Bannister, GC; Lankester, BJ; Brown, JH; Narendra, G; MacGowan, AP. Penetration of linezolid into bone, fat, muscle and haematoma of patients undergoing routine hip replacement. *J. Antimicrob Chemother*, 2002, 50, 73-77.

Lundin, A; Manguson, A; Axelsson, K; Nilson, O; Samuelsson, L. Corticosteroids preoperatively diminishes damage to the C-fibers in microscopic lumbar disc surgery. *Spine*, 2005, 30, 2362-2367.

Lynch, ME; Clark, AJ; Sawynok, J; Sullivan, MJ (a). Topical 2% amitriptyline and 1% ketamine in neuropathic pain syndromes: a randomized, double-blind, placebo-controlled trial. *Anesthesiology*, 2005,103,140-146.

Lynch, ME; Clark, AJ; Sawynok, J; Sullivan, MJ (b). Topical amitriptyline and ketamine in neuropathic pain syndromes: an open-label study. *J. Pain*, 2005, 6, 644-649.

Ma, K; Jiang, W; Zhou, Q; Du, DP. The efficacy of oxycodone for management of acute pain episodes in chronic neck pain patients. *Int. J. Clin. Pract*, 2007, 62, 241-247.

MacLeod, CM; Bartley, EA; Galante, JO; Friedhoff, LT; Dhruv, R. Aztreonam penetration into synovial fluid and bone. *Antimicrob Agents Chemother*, 1986, 29, 710-712.

Mader, JT; Adams, K; Morrison, L. Comparative evaluation of cefazolin and clindamycin in the treatment of experimental Staphylococcus aureus osteomyelitis in rabbits. *Antimicrob Agents Chemother*, 1989, 33, 1760-1764.

Madhusudan, S; Muthuramalingam, SR; Braybrooke, JP; Wilner, S; Kaur, K; Han, C; Hoare, S; Balkwill, F; Ganesan, TS. Study of etanercept, a tumor necrosis factor-alpha inhibitor, in recurrent ovarian cancer. *J. Clin. Oncol*, 2005, 23, 5950-5959.

Mahwold, ML; Singh, JA, Majeski, P. Opioid use by patients in an orthopedics spine clinc. *Arthritis Rheumatism*, 2005, 52, 312-321.

Makela, M; Heliovaara, M; Sievers, K; Impivaara, O; Knekt, P; Aromaa, A. Prevalence, determinants and consequences of chronic neck pain in Finland. *Am. J. Epidemiol.*, 1991, 134, 1356-1367.

Makowska, A; Panfil, C; Ellrich, J. ATP induces sustained facilitation of craniofacial nociception through P2X receptors on neck muscle nociceptors in mice. *Cephalalgia*, 2006, 26, 697-706.

Malawski, SK; Lukawski, S. Pyogenic infection of the spine. *Clin. Orthop.*, 1991, 272, 58-66.

Malincarne, L; Ghebregzabher, M; Moretti, MV; Egidi, AM; Canovari, B; Tavolieri, G; Francisci, D; Cerulli, G; Baldelli F. Penetration of moxifloxacin into bone in patients undergoing total knee arthroplasty. *J. Antimicrob. Chemother*, 2006, 57, 950-954.

Malmberg, AB; Yaksh, TL (a). Hyperalgesia mediated by spinal glutamate or substance P receptor blocked by spinal cyclooxygenase inhibition. *Science*, 1992, 257(5074), 1276-1279.

Malmberg, AB; Yaksh, TL (b). Antinociceptive actions of spinal antisteroidal anti-inflammatory agents on the formalin test in the rat. *J. Pharmacol Exp. Ther*, 1992, 263, 136-146.

Manchikanti, L. Medicare in interventional pain management: a critical analysis. *Pain Physician*, 2006, 9, 171-198.

Manchikanti, L; Pampati, V; Damron, KS; McManus, CD; Jackson, SD; Barnhill, RC; Martin, JC (a). A randomized, prospective, double-blind, placebo-controlled evaluation of the effect of sedation on diagnostic validity of cervical facet joint pain. *Pain Physician*, 2004, 7, 301-309.

Manchikanti L; Boswell MV; Singh V; Pampati V; Damron KS; Beyer CD (b). Prevalence of facet joint pain in chronic spinal pain of cervical, thoracic, and lumbar regions. *BMC Musculoskelet Disord 2004*; 5: 15.

Manfredi, PL; Herskovitz, S; Folli, F; Pigazzi, A; Swerdlow, ML. Spinal epidural abscess: treatment options. *Eur. Neurol.*, 1998, 40, 58-60.

Mantyh, PW; DeMaster, E; Malhotra, A; Ghilardi, JR; Rogers, SD; Mantyh, CR; Liu, H; Basbaum, AI; Vigna, SR; Maggio, JE. Receptor endocytosis and dendrite reshaping in spinal neurons after somatosensory stimulation. *Science*, 1995, 268 (5217), 1629-1632.

Mantyh, PW; Rogers, SD; Honore, P; Allen, BJ; Ghilardi, JR; Li, J; Daughters, RS; Lappi, DA; Wiley, RG; Simone, DA. Inhibition of hyperalgesia by ablation of lamina I spinal neurons expressing the substance P receptor. *Science*, 1997, 278(5336), 275-279.

Mansour, A; Burke, S; Pavlic, RJ; Akil, H; Watson, SJ. Immunohistochemical localization of the cloned kappa 1 receptor in the rat CNS and pituitary. *Neuroscience*, 1996, 71, 671-690.

Mao, J. Translational pain research: bridging the gap between basic and clinical research. *Pain*, 2002, 97, 183–187.

Marchand, F; Tsantoulas, C; Singh, D; Grist, J; Clark, AK; Bradbury, EJ; McMahon, SB. Effects of Etanercept and Minocycline in a rat model of spinal cord injury. *Eur. J. Pain*, 2008, Oct 10.

Marcouiller, P; Pelletier, JP; Guévremont, M; Martel-Pelletier, J; Ranger, P; Laufer, S; Reboul, P. Leukotriene and prostaglandin synthesis pathways in osteoarthritic synovial membranes: regulating factors for interleukin 1beta synthesis. *J. Rheumatol*, 2005, 32, 704-712.

Marienfeld, R; Neumann, M; Chuvpilo, S; Escher, C; Kneitz, B; Avots, A; Schimpl, A; Serfling, E. Cyclosporin A interferes with inducible degradation of NF-kB inhibitors but not with the processing of p105/NF-kB1 in T cells. *Eur. J. Immunol* 1997, 27, 1601-1609.

Marroni, M; Tinca, M; Belfiori, B; Altobelli, G; Malincarne, L; Papili, R; Stagni, G. Nosocomial spondylodiskitis with epidural abscess and liquoral fistula cured with quinupristin/dalfopristin and linezolid. *Infez Med*, 2006, 14, 99-101.

Martin, RJ; Yuan, HA. Neurosurgical care of spinal epidural, subdural, and intramedullary abscesses and arachnoiditis. *Orthop Clin. North Am.*, 1996, 27, 125-136.

Martin, TJ; Eisenach, JC; Misler, J; Childers, SR. Chronic activation of spinal adenosine A1 receptors results in hypersensitivity. *Neuroreport*, 2006, 17, 1619-1622.

Martinez, JH; Mondragon, CE; Céspedes, A. An evaluation of the antiinflammatory effects of intraarticular synthetic β-endorphin in the canine model. *Anesth Analg*, 1996, 82, 177-181.

Matsuki, A. Nothing new under the sun—a Japanese pioneer in the clinical use of intrathecal morphine. *Anesthesiology* 1983, 58, 289-290.

McCarthy, GM; Kenny, D. Dietary fish oil and rheumatic diseases. *Semin Arthritis Rheum*, 1992, 21, 368-375.

McCarthy, DJ; Csuka, M; McCarthy, G; Trotter, D. Treatment of pain due to fibromyalgia with topical capsaicin: a pilot study. *Semin Arthritis Rheum*, 1994, 23(suppl 3), 41-47.

McCleane, GJ (a). Topical doxepin hydrochloride reduces neuropathic pain: a randomized, double-blind, placebo controlled study. *Pain Clin.*, 2000, 12, 47–50.

McCleane, GJ (b). Topical application of doxepin hydrochloride, capsaicin and a combination of both produces analgesia in chronic human neuropathic pain: a randomized, double-blind, placebo-controlled study. *Br. J. Clin. Pharmacol*, 2000, 49, 574–579.

McCormack K. The spinal action of nonsteroidal anti-inflammatory drugs and the dissociation between their anti-inflammatory and analgesic effects. *Drugs* 1994, 47(Suppl 5), 28-45; Discussion 46-47.

McCormack, K; Kidd, BL; Morris, V. Assay of topically administered ibuprofen using a model of post-injury hypersensitivity. A randomised, double-blind, placebo-controlled study. *Eur. J. Clin. Pharmacol*, 2000, 56(6-7), 459-462.

McDougall, JJ; Hanesch, U; Pawlak, M; Schmidt, RF. Participation of NK1 receptors in nociceptin-induced modulation of rat knee joint mechanosensitivity. *Exp. Brain Res*, 2001, 137, 249-253.

McDougall, JJ; Watkins, L; Li, Z .Vasoactive intestinal peptide (VIP) is a modulator of joint pain in a rat model of osteoarthritis. *Pain*, 2006, 123(1-2), 98-105.

McHenry, MC; Easley, KA; Locker, GA. Vertebral osteomyelitis: long-term outcome for 253 patients from 7 Cleveland-area hospitals. *Clin Infect Dis*, 2002, 34, 1342-1350.

McMillan, A; Nolan, A; Kelly, P. The efficacy of dry needling and procaine in the treatment of myofascial pain in the jaw muscles. *J. Orof Pain*, 1997, 11, 307-314.

Merskey, H; Watson, GD. The lateralisation of pain. *Pain*, 1979, 7, 271-280.

Michael, GJ; Averill, S; Nitkunan, A; Rattray, M; Bennett, DL; Yan, Q; Priestley, JV. Nerve growth factor treatment increases brain-derived neurotrophic factor selectively in TrkA-expressing dorsal root ganglion cells and in their central terminations within the spinal cord. *J Neurosci*, 1997, 17, 8476–8490.

Miljanich, GP; Ramachandran, J. Antagonists of neuronal calcium channels: structure, function, and therapeutic implications. *Annu Rev. Pharmacol Toxicol*. 1995, 35, 707-734.

Mironer, EY; Haasis, JC; Chapple, I; Brown, C; Satterthwaite, JR. Efficacy and safety of intrathecal opioid/bupivacaine mixture in chronic nonmalignant pain: A double blind, randomized, crossover, multicenter study by the National Forum of Independent Pain Clinicians (NFIPC). *Neuromodulation*, 2002, 5, 208-213.

Mollenholt, P; Post, C; Rawal, N; Freedman, J; Hökfelt, T; Paulsson, I. Antinociceptive and 'neurotoxic' actions of somatostatin in rat spinal cord after intrathecal administration. *Pain*, 1988, 32, 95-105.

Molloy, RE; Benzon, HT. Interlaminar epidural steroid injections for lumbosacral radiculopathy. In: Benzon HT, Raja SN, Molloy RE, Liu SS, Fishman SM, editors. *Essentials of Pain Medicine and Regional Anesthesia*. Philadelphia, PA: Elsevier Churchill Livingstone; 2005; 331–340.

Moore, RA; Tramèr, MR; Carroll, D; Wiffen, PJ; McQuay, HJ. Quantitative systematic review of topically applied non-steroidal anti-inflammatory drugs. *BMJ*, 1998, 316(7128), 333-338.

Moriya, M; Kimura, T;Yamamoto,Y; Abe, K; Sakoda, S. Successful treatment of cervical spinal epidural abscess without surgery. *Intern Med*, 2005, 44, 1110.

Morton, CR; Hutichson, WD; Hendry, IA. Release of immunoreactive somatostatin in the spinal dorsal horn of the cat. *Neuropeptides*, 1988, 12, 189-197.

Morton, CR; Hutichson, WD. Release of sensory neuropeptides in the spinal cord: Studies with calcitonin gene related peptide and galanin. *Neuroscience*, 1989, 31, 807-815.

Muller, JL; Clauson, KA. Pharmaceutical considerations of common herbal medicine. *Am J Manag Care*, 1997, 3, 1753-1770.

Muller, R; Giles, LG. Long-term follow-up of a randomized clinical trial assessing the efficacy of medication, acupuncture, and spinal manipulation for chronic mechanical spinal pain syndromes. *J. Manipulative Physiol. Ther*, 2005, 28, 3-11.

Müller, J; Kemmler, G; Wissel, J; Schneider, A; Voller, B; Grossmann, J; Diez, J; Homann, N; Wenning, GK; Schnider, P; Poewe, W. The impact of blepharospasm and cervical dystonia on health-related quality of life and depression. *J. Neurol.*, 2002, 249, 842-846.

Murga, G; Samsó, E; Valles, J; Casanovas, P; Puig, MM. The effect of clonidine on intra-operative requirements of fentanyl during combined epidural/general anaesthesia. *Anaesthesia*, 1994, 49, 999-1002.

Muro, K; O'shaughnessy, B; Ganju, A. Infarction of the cervical spinal cord following multilevel transforaminal epidural steroid injection: case report and review of the literature. *J. Spinal Cord Med*, 2007, 30, 385–388.

Naguib, M; Yaksh, TL. Antinociceptive effects of spinal cholinesterase inhibition and isobolographica. *Anesthesiology*, 1994, 80, 1338-1348.

Nagy, JI; Van Der Kooy, D. Effects on neonatal capsaicin treatment on nociceptive thresholds in the rat. *J. Neurosci.*, 1983, 3, 1145-1150.

Nakagawa, T; Wakamatsu, K; Zhang, N; Maeda, S; Minami, M; Satoh, M; Kaneko, S. Intrathecal administration of ATP produces long-lasting allodynia in rats: differential mechanisms in the phase of the induction and maintenance. *Neuroscience*, 2007, 147, 445-455.

Najm, WI; Reinsch, S; Hoehler F, Tobis, JS; Harvey, PW. S-Adenosylmethionine (SAMe) versus celecoxibfor the treatment of osteoarthritissymptoms: A double-blind-cross-over trial. *BMC Musculoskeletal Disorders*, 2004, 5, 6.

Nallu, R; Radhakrishnan, R. Spinal release of acetylcholine in response to morphine. *J. Pain*, 2007, 8, S19.

Neame, R; Zhang, W; Doherty, M. A historic issue of the Annals: three papers examine paracetamol in osteoarthritis. *Ann. Rheum. Dis.* 2004, 63, 897-900.

Neugebauer, V; Rümenapp, P; Schaible, HG. Calcitonin gene-related peptide is involved in the spinal processing of mechanosensory input from the rat's knee joint and in the generation and maintenance of hyperexcitability of dorsal horn-neurons during development of acute inflammation. *Neuroscience*, 1996, 71, 1095-1109.

Nicholas, P; Meyers, BR; Levy, RN; Hirschman, SZ. Concentration of clindamycin in human bone. *Antimicrob Agents Chemother*, 1975, 8, 220-221.

Norimoto, M; Ohtori, S; Yamashita, M; Inoue, G; Yamauchi, K; Koshi, T; Suzuki, M; Orita, S; Eguchi, Y; Sugiura, A; Ochiai, N; Takaso, M; Takahashi, K. Direct application of the TNF-alpha inhibitor, etanercept, does not affect CGRP expression and phenotypic change of DRG neurons following application of nucleus pulposus onto injured sciatic nerves in rats. *Spine*, 2008, 33, 2403-2408.

Nozaki-Taguchi, N; Yaksh, TL. Characterization of the antihyperalgesic action of a novel peripheral mu-opioid receptor agonist--loperamide. *Anesthesiology*, 1999, 90, 225-234.

Oatway, M; Reid, A; Sawynok, J; Peripheral antihyperalgesic and analgesic actions of ketamine and amitriptyline in a model of mild thermal injury in the rat. *Anesth Analg*, 2003, 97, 168-173.

Ojala, T; Arokoski, P; Partanen, J. The effect of small doses of botulinium toxin on a neck shoulder myofacial pain syndrome. A double blind randomized, and controlled crossover trial. *Clin. J. Pain*, 2006, 22, 90-96.

Oku, R; Satoh, M; Fujii, N; Otaka, A; Yajima, H; Takagi, H. calcitonon gene related peptide promotes mechanical nociception by potentiating releaseof substance P from the spinal dorsal horn in rats. *Brain Res.*, 1987, 403, 350-354.

Olesen, J; Diener, H-C; Husstedt, IW; Godasby, PJ; Hall, D; Meier, U; Pollentier, S; Lesko, LM. Calcitonin gene-related peptide (CGRP) receptor antagonist BIBN4096BS for the acute treatment of migraine. *N. Engl. J. Med.*, 2004, 350, 1104–1110.

Olivera, B; Gray, WR; Zeikus, R; McIntosh, JM; Varga, J; Rivier, J;, deSantos, V; Cruz, LJ. Peptide neurotoxins from fish-hunting cone snails. *Science*, 1985, 230, 1338-1343.

Olivera, BM; Cruz, LJ; de Santos, V; LeCheminant, GW; Griffin, D; Zeikus, R; McIntosh, JM; Galyean, R; Varga, J; Gray, WR; et al. Neuronal calcium channel antagonists. Discrimination between calcium channel subtypes using omega-conotoxin from Conus magus venom. *Biochemistry*, 1987, 26, 2086-2090.

Ossipov, MH; Bazov, I; Gardell, LR; Kowal, J; Yakovleva, T; Usynin, I; Ekström, TJ; Porreca, F; Bakalkin, G. Control of chronic pain by the ubiquitin proteasome system in the spinal cord. *J. Neurosci.*, 2007, 27, 8226-8237.

Osti, OL; Fraser, RD; Vernon-Roberts, B. Discitis after discography. The role of prophylactic antibiotics. *J. Bone Joint Surg Br*, 1990, 72, 271-274.

Paliwal, S; Sundaram, J; Mitragotri, S. Induction of cancer-specific cytotoxicity towards human prostate and skin cells using quercetin and ultrasound. *Br. J. Cancer*, 2005, 92, 499-502.

Pan, HL; Khan, GM; Alloway, KD; Chen, SR. Resiniferatoxin induces paradoxical changes in thermal and mechanical sensitivities in rats: mechanism of action. *J. Neurosci.* 2003, 23, 2911–2919.

Paoloni, JA; Appleyard, RC; Nelson, J; Murrell, GA. Topical Nitric Oxide Application in the Treatment of Chronic Extensor Tendinosis at the Elbow. A Randomized, Double-Blinded, Placebo-Controlled Clinical Trial. *The American Journal of Sports Medicine*, 2003, 31, 915-920.

Park, JY; Jun, IG. The interaction of gabapentin and N6-(2-phenylisopropyl)-adenosine R-(-)isomer (R-PIA) on mechanical allodynia in rats with a spinal nerve ligation. *J Korean Med Sci,* 2008, 23, 678-684.

Paulose-Ram, R; Hirsch, R; Dillon, C; Gu, Q. Frequent monthly use of selected non-prescription and prescription non-narcotic analgesics among U.S. adults. *Pharmacoepidemiol Drug Saf*, 2005, 14, 257-266.

Pavelka, K; Gatterova, J; Olejarova, M; Machacek, S; Giacovelli, G; Rovati, LC. Glucosamine sulfate use and delay of progression of knee osteoarthritis: a 3-year, randomized, placebo-controlled, double-blind study. *Arch. Intern. Med.*, 2002, 162, 2113-2123.

Pederson, JL; Galle, TS; Kehlet, H. Peripheral analgesic effects of ketamine in acute inflammatory pain. *Anesthesiology,* 1998, 89, 58-66.

Penerai, AE; Massei, R; DeSilva, G; Sacerdote, P; Monza, G; mantegazza, P. Baclofen prolongs the analgesic effect of fentanyl in man. *British Journal of Anaesthesia* 1985, 57, 954-955.

Pert, CB; Snyder, S. Opiate receptor: Demonstration in nervous tissue. *Science*, 1973, 179, 1011-1014.

Pertwee, RG. Cannabinoid receptors and pain..*Prog. Neurobiol.*, 2001, 63, 569-611.

Picavet, HS; Schouten, JS: Musculoskeletal pain in the Netherlands: prevalences, consequences and risk groups, the DMC(3)-study. *Pain*, 2003, 102(1–2), 167-178.

Pincus, T; Koch, G; Lei, H; Mangal, B; Sokka, T; Moskowitz, R; Wolfe, F; Gibofsky, A; Simon,L; Zlotnick, S; Fort, JG. Patient Preference for Placebo, Acetaminophen (paracetamol) or Celecoxib Efficacy Studies (PACES): two randomised, double blind, placebo controlled, crossover clinical trials in patients with knee or hip osteoarthritis. *Ann. Rheum Dis.*, 2004, 63, 931-939.

Pini, LA; Sandrini, M; Vitale, G. The antinociceptive action of paracetamol is associated with changes in the serotonergic system in the rat brain. *Eur. J. Pharmacol*, 1996, 308, 31-40.

Podichetty,VK. The aging spine: the role of inflammatory mediators in intervertebral disc degeneration. *Cell Mol. Biol.*, 2007, 53, 4-18.

Pohl, M; Lombard, MC; Bourgoin, S; Carayon, A; Benoliel, JJ; Mauborgne, A; Besson, JM; Cesselin, F. Opioid control of the in vitro release of calcitonin gene-related peptide from primary afferent fibres projecting in the rat cervical cord. *Neuropeptides,* 1989, 14, 151–159.

Post, C; Alari, L; Hökfelt, T. Intrathecal galanin increases the latency in the tail-flick and hot-plate test in mouse. *Acta Physiol. Scand*, 1988, 132, 583-584.

Prado, WA; Dias, TB. Postoperative Analgesia Induced by Intrathecal Neostigmine or Bethanechol in Rats. *Clin. Exp. Pharmacol. Physiol.*, 2008 Nov 28.

Qerama, E; Fugisang-Frederiksen, A; Kasch , H; Bach, FW; Jensen, TS. A double blind controlled study of botulinium toxin A in chronic myofacial pain. *Neurology*, 2006, 67, 241-245.

Qinyang, W; Hultenby, K; Adlan, E; Lindgren, JU. Galanin in adjuvant arthritis in the rat. *J. Rheumatol*, 2004, 31, 302-307.

Radhakrishnan, V; Henry, JL. Electrophysiology of neuropeptides in the sensory spinal cord. *Prog. Brain Res.*, 1995, 104, 175-195.

Rahme, E; Barkun, A; Nedjar, H; Gaugris, S; Watson, D. Hospitalizations for upper and lower GI events associated with traditional NSAIDs and acetaminophen among the elderly in Quebec, Canada. *Am. J. Gastroenterol*, 2008, 103, 872-882.

Rao, SG. The neuropharmacology of centrally-acting analgesic medications in fibromyalgia. *Rheum Dis. Clin. North Am.*, 2002, 28, 235-259.

Recommendations for the medical management of osteoarthritis of the hip and knee: 2000 update. American College of Rheumatology Subcommittee on Osteoarthritis Guidelines. *Arthritis Rheum*, 2000, 43, 1905-1915.

Reeves, KD. Prolotherapy: Present and Future Applications in Soft-Tissue Pain and Disability. Injection Techniques: Principles and Practice. *Physical Medicine and Rehabilitation Clinics of North America,* 1995, 4, 917-923.

Reeves, KD. Prolotherapy: Basic Science, Clinical Studies, and Technique. In: Lennard TA (Ed): *Pain Procedures in Clinical Practice*, 2nd edition. Philadelphia; Hanley and Belfus; 2000; 172-190.

Reginster, JY; Deroisy, R; Rovati, LC; Lee, RL; Lejeune, E; Bruyere, O; Giacovelli, G; Henrotin, Y; Dacre, JE; Gossett, C. Long-term effects of glucosamine sulphate on osteoarthritis progression: a randomised, placebo-controlled clinical trial. *Lancet*, 2001, 357, 251-256.

Reynolds, IJ; Miller, RJ. Tricyclic antidepressants block N-methyl-D-aspartate receptors: similarities to the action of zinc. *Br. J. Pharmacol.* 1988, 95, 95–102.

Rezai, M; Côté, P; Cassidy, JD; Carroll, L. The association between prevalent neck pain and health-related quality of life: a cross-sectional analysis. *Eur. Spine J.*, 2008 Nov 20.

Rhoten, RLP; Murphy, MA; Kalfas, IH; Hahn, JF; Washington, JA. Antibiotic penetration into cervical discs. *Neurosurgery*, 1995, 37, 418-421.

Richardson, BP; Engel, G; Donatsch, P; Stadler, PA. Identification of serotonin M-receptor subtypes and their specific blockade by a new class of drugs. *Nature*, 1985, 316 (6024), 126-131.

Richy, F; Bruyere, O; Ethgen, O; Cucherat, M; Henrotin, Y; Reginster, J-Y. Structural and symptomatic efficacy of glucosamine and chondroitin in knee osteoarthritis. A comprehensive meta-analysis. *Arch. Intern. Med.*, 2003, 163, 1514-1522.

Rimmelé, T; Boselli, E; Breilh, D; Djabarouti, S; Bel, JC; Guyot, R; Saux, MC; Allaouchiche, B. Diffusion of levofloxacin into bone and synovial tissues. *J. Antimicrob Chemother*, 2004; 53: 533-535.

Rosomoff, HL; Fishbain, DA; Goldberg, M; Santana, R; Rosomoff, RS. Physical findings in patients with chronic intractable benign pain of the neck and/or back. *Pain*, 1989, 37, 279-287.

Rowlingson, JC; Kirschenbaum, LP. Epidural analgesic techniques in the management of cervical pain. *Anesth Analg*, 1986, 65, 938-942.

Ruan, X. Drug-related side effects of long-term intrathecal morphine therapy: A focused review. *Pain Physician*, 2007, 10, 357-366.

Rueff, A; Dray, A. Pharmacological characterization of the effects of 5-hydroxytryptamine and different prostaglandins on peripheral sensory neurons in vitro. *Agents Actions*, 1993, C13-15.

Ryöppy, S; Jääskeläinen, J; Rapola, J; Alberty, A. Nonspecific diskitis in children. A nonmicrobial disease? *Clin. Orthop*,1993, 297, 95-99.

Salonen, MA; Kanto, JH; Maze, M. Clinical interactions with alpha-2-adrenergic agonists in anesthetic practice. *J. Clin. Anesth*, 1992, 4, 164-172.

Sang, C; Jenkins, K; Wang, K; Sarin, A; Coccoli, S. Fosphenytoin relieves neuropathic pain following spinal cord injury. *Program and abstracts of the 25th Annual Scientific Meeting of the American Pain Society*; May 3-6, 2006; San Antonio, Texas. Poster 692.

Sano, T; Sakurai, M; Dohi, S; Oyama,A; Murota, K; Sugiyama, H; Miura, Y; Kusuoka, K; Kurata, K. Investigation of meropenem levels in the human bone marrow blood, bone, joint fluid and joint tissues. *Jpn J. Antibiot*, 1993, 46,159-163.

Sapico, FL: Microbiology and antimicrobial therapy of spinal infections. *Orthop Clin. North Am.*, 1996, 27, 9-13.

Sapico, FL; Montgomerie, JZ. Pyogenic vertebral osteomyelitis: re port of nine cases and review of the literature. *Rev. Infect Dis.*, 1979, 1,754-776.

Sastravaha, G; Gassman, G; Sangtherapitikul, P; Grimm, WD. Adjunctive periodontal therapy with Centella asiatica and Punica granatum extracts in supportive periodontal therapy. *J. Int Acad Periodontl*, 2005, 7, 70-79.

Sawynok J, Sweeney MI. The role of purines in nociception. *Neuroscience*, 1989, 32, 557–569.

Schellingerhout, JM; Verhagen, AP; Heymans, MW; Pool, JJ; Vonk, F; Koes, BW; de Vet, HC. Which subgroups of patients with non-specific neck pain are more likely to benefit from spinal manipulation therapy, physiotherapy, or usual care? *Pain*, 2008, Sep 4.

Schimmer, RC; Jeanneret, C; Nunley, PD; Jeanneret, B. Osteomyelitis of the cervical spine: a potentially dramatic disease. *J. Spinal Disord Tech.*, 2002, 15, 110-117.

Schreiber, AL; Formal, CS. Spinal cord infarction secondary to cocaine use. *Am. J. Phys. Med. Rehabil*, 2007, 86, 158-160.

Schurman, DJ; Burton, DS; Kajiyama, G. Cefoxitin antibiotic concentration in bone and synovial fluid. *Clin. Orthop Relat Res.*, 1982, 168, 64-68.

Schofferman, J. Long-term use of opioid analgesics for the treatment of chronic pain of nonmalignant origin. *J. Pain Symptom Manage*, 1993, 8, 279-288.

Scuderi, GJ; Greenberg, SS; Banovac, K; Martinez, OV; Eismont, FJ. Penetration of glycopeptide antibiotics in nucleus pulposus. *Spine*, 1993, 14, 2039-2042

See, S; Ginsburg, R. Choosing a skeletal muscle relaxant. *Am. Fam Physician*, 2008, 78, 365-370.

Serhan, CN. Lipoxins and aspirin-triggered 15-epi-lipoxins are the first lipid mediators of endogenous anti-inflammation and resolution. *Prostaglandins Leukot Essent Fatty Acids*, 2005, 73(3-4), 141-162.

Serhan, CN. Resolution phase of inflammation: novel endogenous anti-inflammatory and proresolving lipid mediators and pathways. *Annu. Rev. Immunol.*, 2007, 25, 101–137.

Serhan, CN; Chiang, N; Van Dyke, TE. Resolving inflammation: dual anti-inflammatory and pro-resolution lipid mediators. *Nat. Rev. Immunol*, 2008, 8, 349-361.

Serhan, CN; Hamberg, M; Samuelsson, B. Lipoxins: novel series of biologically active compounds formed from arachidonic acid in human leukocytes. *Proc. Natl. Acad. Sci. USA*, 1984, 81, 5335-5339.

Serhan, CN; Hong, S; Gronert, K; Colgan, SP; Devchand, PR; Mirick, G; Moussignac, RL. Resolvins: a family of bioactive products of omega-3 fatty acid transformation circuits initiated by aspirin treatment that counter proinflammation signals. *J. Exp. Med.*, 2002, 196, 1025-1037.

Serhan, C N; Savill, J. Resolution of inflammation: the beginning programs the end. *Nature Immunol*, 2005, 6, 1191–1197.

Sekiguchi, M; Shirasaka, M; Konno, S-I; Kikuchi, S. Analgesic effect of percutaneously absorbed non-steroidal anti-inflammatory drugs: an experimental study in a rat acute inflammation model. *BMC Muscloskeletal Disoredrs*, 2008, 9, 15.

Sharma, S; Chopra, K; Kulkarni, SK. Effect of insulin and its combination with resveratrol or curcumin in attenuation of diabetic neuropathic pain: participation of nitric oxide and TNF-alpha. *Phytother Res*, 2007, 147, 155-163.

Shen, CL; Hong, KJ; Kim, SW. Comparative effects of ginger root (Zingiber officinale Rosc.) on the production of inflammatory mediators in normal and osteoarthrotic sow chondrocytes. *J. Med. Food*, 2005, 8, 149-153.

Sherman, KJ; Cherkin, DC; Erro, J; Hrbek, A; Eisenberg, DM; Davis, RB. The diagnosis and treatment of chronic back pain by acupuncturist, chiropractors and massage therapists. *Clin. J. Pain*, 2006, 22, 227-234.

Shukla M, Gupta K, Rasheed Z, Khan KA, Haqqi TM. Bioavailable constituents/ metabolites of pomegranate (*Punica granatum* L) preferentially inhibit COX2 activity *ex vivo* and IL-

1beta-induced PGE2 production in human chondrocytes *in vitro. Journal of Inflammation*, 2008, 5:9 doi:10.1186/1476-9255-5-9.

Siddall, PJ; Molloy, AR; Walker, S; Mather, LE; Rutkowski, SB; Cousins, MJ. The efficacy of intrathecal morphine and clonidine in the treatment of pain after spinal cord injury. *Anesth. Analg*, 2000, 91, 1493-1498.

Singh, G; Shetty, RR; Ramdass, MJ; Ravidass, MJ; Anilkumar, PG. Cervical osteomyelitis associated with intravenous drug use. *Emerg Med. J.*, 2006, 23, e16.

Sjölund, K-F; von Hejne, M; Hao, J-X. Intrathecal administration of the adenosine A1 receptor agonist R-phenylisopropyl adenosine reduces presumed pain behaviour in a rat model of central pain. *Neurosci. Lett*, 1998, 243, 89–92.

Sodin-Semrl, S; Spagnolo, A; Barbaro, B; Varga, J; Fiore, S. Lipoxin A4 counteracts synergistic activation of human fibroblast-like synoviocytes. *Int. J. Immunopathol Pharmacol.*, 2004, 17, 15-25.

Sodin-Semrl, S; Taddeo, B; Tseng, D; Varga, J; Fiore, S. Lipoxin A4 inhibits IL-1 beta-induced IL-6, IL-8, and matrix metalloproteinase-3 production in human synovial fibroblasts and enhances synthesis of tissue inhibitors of metalloproteinases. *J. Immunol.*, 2000, 164, 2660-2666.

Simone, DA; Alreja, M; LaMotte, RH. Psychophysical studies of the itch sensation and itchy skin ("alloknesis") produced by intracutaneous injection of histamine. *Somatosens Mot Res*, 1991, 8, 271-279.

Simons, DG; Travell, JG; Simons, LS. Travell and Simons' Myofascial Pain and Dysfunction: The Trigger Point Manual. 2nd edition. Baltimore: Williams and Wilkins; 2002.

Simons, DG: Fibrositis/fibromyalgia: a form of myofascial trigger points? *Am. J. Med.*, 1986, 81, 93-98.

Singh, J; Budhiraja, S. Therapeutic potential of cannabinoid receptor ligands: current status. *Methods Find Exp. Clin. Pharmacol*, 2006, 28, 177-183.

Sist, T; Miner, M; Lema, M. Characteristics of postradical neck pain syndrome: a report of 25 cases. *J. Pain Symptom. Manage*, 1999, 18, 95-102.

Slipman, CW; Lipetz, JS; Jackson, HB; Rogers, DP; Vresilovic, EJ. Therapeutic selective nerve root block in the nonsurgical treatment of atraumatic cervical spondylotic radicular pain: a retrospective analysis with independent clinical review. *Arch. Phys. Med. Rehabil*, 2000; 81:741–746.

Solomou, E; Maragkos, M; Kotsarini, C; Konstantinou, D; Maraziotis, T. Multiple spinal epidural abscesses extending to the whole spinal canal. *Magn Reson Imaging* 2004, 22, 747-750.

Staats, PS; Yearwood, T; Charapata, SG; Presley, RW; Wallace, MS; Byas-Smith, M; Fisher, R; Bryce, DA; Mangieri, EA; Luther, RR; Mayo, M; McGuire, D; Ellis, D. Intrathecal ziconotide in the treatment of refractory pain in patients with cancer or AIDS: A randomized controlled trial. *JAMA*, 2004, 291, 63-70.

Steen, AE; Reeh, PW; Geisslinger, G; Steen, KH. Plasma levels after peroral and topical ibuprofen and effects upon low pH-induced cutaneous and muscle pain. *Eur. J. Pain*, 2000, 4, 195-209.

Stein, C; Yassouridis A. Peripheral morphine analgesia. *Pain*, 1997; 71(2):119-121.

Suzuki, N; Hardebo, JE; Owman, C. Trigeminal fibre collaterals storing substance P and calcitonin gene-related peptide associate with ganglion cells containing choline acetyltransferase and vasoactive intestinal polypeptide in the sphenopalatine ganglion of the rat. An axon reflex modulating parasympathetic ganglionic activity? *Neuroscience,* 1989, 30, 595-604.

Svensson, CI; Zattoni, M; Serhan, CN. Lipoxins and aspirin-triggered lipoxins inhibit inflammatory pain processing. *J. Exp. Med.,* 2007, 204, 245-252.

Sycha T, Kranz G, Auff E, Schnider P. Botulinum toxin in the treatment of rare head and neck pain syndromes: a systematic review of the literature. *J. Neurol.,* 2004, Feb, I19-30.

Szallasi, A; Blumberg, PM; Annicelli, LL; Krause, JE; Cortright, DN. The cloned rat vanilloid receptor VR1 mediates both R-type binding and C-type calcium response in dorsal root ganglion neurons. *Mol. Pharmacol.,* 1999, 56, 581–587.

Szallasi, A. Vanilloid receptor ligands: hopes and realities for the future. *Drugs Aging,* 2001, 18, 561–573.

Tai, CC; Want, S; Quraishi, NA; Batten, J; Kalra, J; Hughes, SPF. Antibiotic prophylaxis in surgery of the intervertebral disc: A comparison between gentamicin and cefuroxime. *J Bone Joint Surg [Br],* 2002, 84-B, 1036-1039.

Taiwo YO, Levine JD. Kappa- and delta-opioids block sympathetically dependent hyperalgesia. *J. Neurosci.,* 1991, 11, 928-932.

Tal, M; Bennett, GJ. Dextrorphan relieves neuropathic heat-evoked hyperalgesia in the rat. *Neurosci. Lett,* 1993, 141, 107–110.

Tandon, N; Vollmer, DG. Infections of the spine and spinal cord. In:Winn HR (ed). *Youmans Neurological Surgery,* edition 5. Philadelphia: Saunders; 2004; Vol 4; pp; 4363-4394.

Taricco, M; Pagliacci, MC; Telaro, E; Adone, R. Pharmacological interventions for spasticity following spinal cord injury: Results of a Cochrane systematic review. *Eura Medicophys,* 2006, 42, 5-15.

Tarsy, D. Comparison of acute- and delayed-onset posttraumatic cervical dystonia. *Mov. Disord.,* 1998, 13, 481-485.

Taylor, HH; Murphy, B. Altered sensorimotor integration with cervical spine manipulation. *J. Manipulative Physiol. Ther,* 2008, 31, 115-126.

Terenius, L. Characteristics of the "receptor" for narcotic analgesics in synaptic plasma membrane fractions from rat brain. *Acta Pharmacol Toxicol.,* 1973, 33, 377-384.

Uchida, S; Hirai, K; Hatanaka, J; Hanato, J; Umegaki, K; Yamada, S. Antinociceptive Effects of St. John's Wort, Harpagophytum Procumbens Extract and Grape Seed Proanthocyanidins Extract in Mice. *Biol. Pharm. Bull,* 2008, 31, 240-245.

Tzchentke, TM; De Vry, J; Christoph, T et al. Tapentadol HCl: analgesic profile of a novel centrally active analgesic with dual mode of action in animal models of nociception, inflammatory and neuropathic pain. *Program and abstracts of the 25th Annual Scientific Meeting of the American Pain Society;* May 3-6, 2006; San Antonio, Texas. Poster 687.

Uhle, EI; Becker, R; Gatscher, S; Bertalanffy, H. Continuous intrathecal clonidine administration for the treatment of neuropathic pain. *Stereotact Funct Neurosurg,* 2000, 75, 167-175.

Urban, L; Thompson, SW; Dray, A. Modulation of spinal excitability: co-operation between neurokinin and excitatory amino acid neurotransmitters. *Trends Neurosci.,* 1994, 17, 432-438.

Usha, PR; Naidu, MUR. Randomised, double-blind, parallel, placebo-controlled study of oral glucosamine, methylsulfonylmethane and their combination in osteoarthritis. *Clin. Drug Invest,* 2004, 24, 353–363.

Vaile, JH; Davis, P. Topical NSAIDs for musculoskeletal conditions. A review of the literature. *Drugs*, 1998, 56, 783-799.

van der Velde, G; Hogg-Johnson, S; Bayoumi, AM; Cassidy, JD; Côté, P; Boyle, E; Llewellyn-Thomas, H; Chan, S; Subrata, P; Hoving, JL; Hurwitz, E; Bombardier, C; Krahn, M. Identifying the best treatment among common nonsurgical neck pain treatments: a decision analysis. *Spine*, 2008, 33(4 Suppl), S184-191.

van Dongen, RT; Crul, BJ; van Egmond, J. Intrathecal coadministration of bupivacaine diminishes morphine dose progression during long-term intrathecal infusion in cancer patients. *Clin. J. Pain*, 1999; 15:166-172.

van Hilten; BJ; van de Beek, WJ; Hoff, JI; Voormolen, JH; Delhaas, EM. Intrathecal baclofen for the treatment of dystonia in patients with reflex sympathetic dystrophy. *N. Engl. J. Med.*, 2000, 343,625-630.

Van Tulder, MW; Touray, T; Furla, AD; Solway, S; Bouter, LM. Muscle relaxants for non-specific low back pain. *Cochrane Database Syst Rev*, 2003, (2): CD004252.doi:10.1002/14651858:CD004252. PMID 12804507.

Vaught, JL. Substance P antagonists and analgesia: a review of the hypothesis. *Life Sci*, 1988, 43, 1419-1431.

Wagner, R; Myers, RR. Endoneurial injection of TNF-alpha produces neuropathic pain behaviors. *Neuroreport*, 1996, 7, 2897-2901.

Waldmann, R; Champigny, G; Bassilana, F; Heurteaux, C; Lazdunski, M. A proton-gated cation channel involved in acid-sensing. *Nature*, 1997, 386(6621), 173-177.

Walid, MS; Hyer, L; Ajjan, M; Barth, AC; Robinson, JS. Prevalence of opioid dependence in spine surgery and correlation with length stay. *J. Opioid Manag*, 2007, 3, 127-128, 130-132.

Wallace, M; Yaksh, TL. Long term spinal analgesic delivery: A review of preclinical and clinical literature. *Reg Anesth Pain Med.*, 2000, 25, 117-157.

Wallin, MK; Raak, RI. Quality of life in subgroups of individuals with whiplash associated disorders.*Eur. J. Pain*, 2008, 12, 842-849.

Walsh, AJ; O'neill, CW; Lotz, JC. Glucosamine HCl alters production of inflammatory mediators by rat intervertebral disc cells in vitro. *Spine J*, 2007, 7, 601-608.

Walters, R; Vernon-Roberts, B; Fraser, R; Moore, R. Therapeutic use of cephazolin to prevent complications of spine surgery. *Inflammopharmacology,* 2006, 14, 138-143.

Wang, SM; Kain, ZN; White, PF. Acupuncture analgesia: II. Clinical considerations. *Anesth Analg*, 2008,106, 611-621.

Warncke, T; Jorum, E; Stubhaug, A. Local treatment with N-methyl-D-aspartate receptor antagonist ketamine, inhibits development of secondary hyperalgesia in man by a peripheral action. *Neurosci Lett*, 1997, 227, 1-4.

Warner, TD; Mitchell, JA. Cyclooxygenase-3 (COX-3): filling in the gaps toward a COX continuum? *Proc Natl Acad Sci USA*, 2002, 99, 13371-13373.

Watson, CPN.Topical capsaicin as an adjuvant analgesic. *J Pain Symptom Manage*, 1994, 9, 425-433.

Watson, CP; Babul, N. Efficacy of oxycodone in neuropathic pain: a randomized trial in post-herpetic neuralgia. *Neurology*, 1998, 50, 1837-1841.

Weisman, H; Hagaman, C; Yaksh, TL; Lotz, M. Preliminaryfindings on the role of neuropeptide suppression bytopical agents in the managementof rheumatoid arthritis. *Seminars in Arthritisand Rheumatism*, 1994, 23 (suppl 3), 18-24.

Welch, SP; Stevens, DL. Antinociceptive activity of intrathecally administered cannabinoids alone, and in combination with morphine, in mice. *J. Pharmacol. Exp. Ther*, 1992, 262, 10-18.

Welch, SP; Singha, AK; Dewey, WL. The antinociception produced by intrathecal morphine, calcium, A23187, U50, 488H, [D-Ala2, N-Me-Phe4, Glyol]enkephalin and [D-Pen2, D-Pen5]enkephalin after intrathecal administration of calcitonin gene-related peptide in mice. *J. Pharmacol. Exp. Ther*, 1989, 251, 1–8.

Wenger, DR; Bobechko, WP; Gilday, DL. The spectrum of intervertebral disc-space infection in children. *J. Bone Joint Surg. Am.*, 1978, 60, 100-108.

White, AR; Ernst, E. A systematic review of randomized controlled trials of acupuncture for neck pain. *Rheumatology*, 1999, 38, 143-147.

Wiech, K; Kiefer, RT; Töpfner, S; Preissl, H; Braun, C; Unertl, K; Flor, H; Birbaumer, N. A placebo-controlled randomized crossover trial of the N-methyl-D-aspartic acid receptor antagonist, memantine, in patients with chronic phantom limb pain. *Anesth Analg*, 2004, 98, 408-413.

Wood, R. Ketamine for pain in hospice patients. *Int. J. Pharm. Compound.*, 2000, 4, 258–259.

Woolf ,CJ; Mannion, RJ. Neuropathic pain: Aetiology, symptoms, mechanisms and management. *Lancet*, 1999, 353, 1959-1964.

Wu, J. Anti-inflammatory ingredients. *J. Drugs Dermatol.*, 2008, 7(7 Suppl), S13-16.

Xu, XJ; Farkas-Szallasi, T; Lundberg, JM Hökfelt, T; Wiesenfeld-Hallin, Z; Szallasi, A . Effects of the capsaicin analogue resiniferatoxin on spinal nociceptive mechanisms in the rat: behavioural, electrophysiological and *in situ* hybridization studies. *Brain Res*, 1997, 752, 52–60.

Yaksh, TL. Behavioral and autonomic correlates of the tactile evoked allodynia produced by spinal glycine inhibition: effects of modulatory receptor systems and excitatory amino acid antagonists. *Pain*, 1989, 37, 111-123.

Yaksh, TL; Dirig, DM; Malmberg, AB. Mechanism of action of nonsteroidal anti-inflammatory drugs. *Cancer Invest*, 1998, 16, 509-527.

Yamauchi ,M; Asano, M; Watanabe, M; Iwasaki,S; Furuse, S; Namiki, A. Continuous dose ketamine improves the analgesic effects of fentanyl patient-controlled analgesia after cervical spine surgery. *Anesth Analg*, 2008, 107, 1041-1041.

Yanagisawa, M; Yagi, N; Otsuka, M; Yanaihara, C; Yanaihara, N. Inhibitory effects of galanin on the isolated spinal cord of the newborn rat. *Neurosci. Lett*, 1986, 70, 278-282.

Yelland, MJ; Nikles, CJ; McNairn, N; Del Mar, CB; Schluter, PJ; Brown, RM. Celecoxib compared with sustained-release paracetamol for osteoarthritis: a series of n-of-1 trials. *Rheumatololgy* (Oxford), 2006, 46, 135-140.

Yu, LC; Lundeberg, S; An, H; Wang, FX; Lundeberg, T. Effects of intrathecal galanin on nociceptive responses in rats with mononeuropathy. *Life Sci.*, 1999, 64, 1145-1153.

Zanella, JM; Burright, EN; Hildebrand, K; Hobot, C; Cox, M; Christoferson, L; McKay, WF. Effect of etanercept, a tumor necrosis factor-alpha inhibitor, on neuropathic pain in the rat chronic constriction injury model. *Spine*, 2008, 33, 227-234.

Zesiewicz, TA; Stamey, W; Sullivan, KL; Hauser, RA. Botulinum toxin A for the treatment of cervical dystonia. *Expert Opin Pharmacother*, 2004, 5, 2017-2024.

Zhang, W; Jones, A; Doherty, M. Does paracetamol (acetaminophen) reduce the pain of osteoarthritis? A meta-analysis of randomised controlled trials. *Ann. Rheum Dis.*, 2004, 63, 901-907.

Zhang, HM; Chen, SR; Cai, YQ; Richardson, TE; Driver, LC; Lopez-Berestein, G; Pan, HL. Signaling mechanisms mediating muscarinic enhancement of GABAERGIC synaptic transmission in the spinal cord. *Neuroscience*, 2008 Dec 7.

Zochodne, DW; Ho, LT. Sumatriptan blocks neurogenic inflammation in the peripheral nerve trunk. *Neurology*, 1994, 44, 161-163.

Zubrzycka, M; Janecka, A; KoziolKiewicz, W; Traczyk, WZ. Inhibition of tongue reflex in rats by tooth pulb stimulation during cerebral ventricle perfusion with (6-11) substance P analogs. *Brain Res.*, 1997, 753,128-132.

Zwart, JA; Dyb, G; Hagen, K; Svebak, S; Holmen, J. Analgesic use: a predictor of chronic pain and medication overuse headache: the Head-HUNT Study. *Neurology*, 2003, 61,160-164.

Zygmunt, PM; Petersson, J; Andersson, DA; Chuang, H; Sørgård, M; Di Marzo, V; Julius, D; Högestätt, ED . Vanilloid receptors on sensory nerves mediate the vasodilator action of anandamide. Nature, 1999, 400 (6743), 452—457.

In: Neck Pain: Causes, Diagnosis and Management
Editor: Gregorio Lombardi

ISBN 978-1-61470-363-1
© 2012 Nova Science Publishers, Inc.

Chapter 7

FEAR-AVOIDANCE BELIEFS-A CHALLENGE TO THE TRADITIONAL DISEASE MODEL FOR TREATMENT OF NECK PAIN

Kwok-Chung Lee and Thomas T. W. Chiu[*]

Department of Rehabilitation Sciences,
the Hong Kong Polytechnic University, China

ABSTRACT

Neck pain is a common symptom in the population. Successful management of neck pain is a real challenge to clinicians. Understanding the pain pathways is essential when investigating pain mechanisms and its management. This article gives a brief review of the pain pathways at the simplest form, leading to the fact that pain can be modulated by the past experiences, emotions and cultural background of the person via sensory-discriminative, cognitive-behavioral and affective-emotional mechanisms.

The traditional Cartesian model of specific pain pathways is deeply rooted in the concepts of the clinical management of patients suffering from pain or disease. However, this traditional management for patients with neck pain, from an evidence-based perspective, is now a point of controversy in the literature. On the contrary, a new trend in considering psychosocial factors in the management of spinal pain had been established. There is increasing evidence to support the belief that the clinical presentation of chronic disability could be better understood and managed by using a biopsychosocial model which, as its name implies, considers the influence and interaction of physical, psychological and social factors on human pain perception and behaviors.

Among the psychosocial factors, the fear-avoidance beliefs as set out in the Fear-Avoidance Beliefs Model developed by Lethem et al. have been hypothesized as one of the most important, specific and powerful cognitive variables in predicting disability and treatment outcome in patients with lower back pain. In a recent study involving 120 patients with chronic neck pain the present authors demonstrate that the fear-avoidance belief is an important measure in addition to pain, physical impairments, disability and health status measures. Moreover, the fear-avoidance belief is an important psychosocial

---

[*] Telephone Number: (852) 27666709, Fax: (852) 23308656, Email: rstchiu@polyu.edu.hk

factor in predicting the level of future disability and the likelihood of return to complete work capacity at the earlier phase of rehabilitation. These findings lend good support to the recommendation that early identification of patients with high fear-avoidance beliefs would help in planning an appropriate treatment for them to prevent the development of chronic disability and incapacity to work, therefore reducing the socioeconomic impact of neck pain to society.

Neck pain is a common symptom in the population. A review of different observational studies of neck pain over the world showed that the one-year prevalence ranged from 16.7% to 75.1% for the entire adult population (17-70 years) with a mean of 37.2%, and the prevalence is independent of age but higher in women than men (Fejer et al. 2006). Neck pain also causes a significant expense in modern society. The total cost of neck pain in the Netherlands in 1996 was about 1% of the total health care expenditure (Borghouts et al.1999). Neck pain is associated with work absenteeism and restricted work duty in nurses, and its social impact included inadequate sleep as well as reduced participation in non-work activities and recreation (Trinkoff et al. 2002). Therefore, neck pain is a global health problem which greatly affects a person's quality of life. Effective management of patients with neck pain continues to be a real challenge to clinicians.

THE DEFINITION AND COMPLEXITY OF PAIN

Understanding the pain pathways first is essential when investigating chronic pain mechanisms. The pain pathways, at the simplest form, consist of three orders or levels of neurons: spinal cord, brainstem, and forebrain.

First-order neurons reside within the dorsal root ganglia (DRG). In the dorsal horn, second-order neurons project and ascend in the spinothalamic tract. It is the first site of synaptic transfer in the nociceptive pathway and is subject to considerable local and descending modulation (Bolay et al. 2002). Plasticity or modifiability of synaptic transfer in the dorsal horn is a key feature of its function and is integral to the generation of pain and pain hypersensitivity. In the dorsal horn, nociception-specific neurons locate in laminae I and II and respond only to noxious inputs and can be sensitized by repetitive stimulation. It is found that somatic and visceral afferents converge on these neurons, thus suggesting a role in pain referral.

Third-order neurons locate in the thalamus and project to the primary somatosensory and cingulate cortices. Noxious stimuli transmit from the periphery to the spinal cord and brainstem through small myelinated A α-fibers and small unmyelinated C-fibers (Patestas and Gartner 2006). After stimulation, high-threshold mechanoreceptors and A α-fibers are recruited initially and transmit the acute local painful stimulus. More intense stimuli, perceived as diffuse, unpleasant, and persistent burning sensations that last beyond the acute painful stimulus and which are slightly delayed in their onset, were activated from polymodal nociceptors. Mechanoreceptors and polymodal nociceptors contain the neurotransmitter l-glutamate, and polymodal nociceptors also contain the neuropeptides substance P, calcitonin gene-related peptide (CGRP), and neurokinin A. The affective and motivational pathways account for dysphoric elements of a noxious experience. It involves structures such as the parabrachial nucleus, amygdala, and intralaminar nucleus of the thalamus (Figure 1.) (Bolay et al. 2002).

The word "pain" is derived from the Latin word "poena" or "dolor", meaning suffering, penalty, grief, misery or punishment (Online English to Latin to English

Dictionary). However, the complexity of pain is much more than these original meanings. This can be easily understood by observing how everyone responds to pain in daily life.

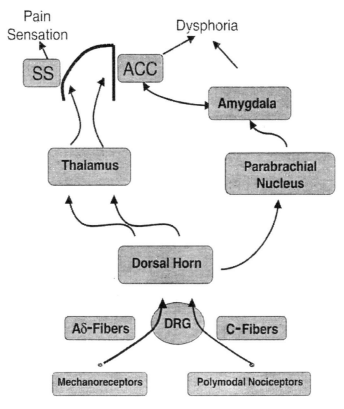

Figure 1. Pain pathways. SS = somatosensory cortex; ACC = anterior cingulate cortex; DRG = dorsal root ganglia (Bolay et al. 2002).

Once the noxious stimulus has been encountered by our body, this noxious stimulus immediate activates specialized motor nerve fibers to send signals to remove the body away from the stimulus through a peripheral reflex loop nerve network. At the same time, the signals continue on to the somatosensory cortex of the brain where it is interpreted as pain and is localized. With the projections to the limbic system via thalamus, the emotional response to the noxious stimulus may be expressed by grimacing, crying, screaming, fear, anxiety or even fainting depending on the cultural or socioeconomic backgrounds in which a person is raised and how that environment deals with pain and responses to pain.

Therefore, pain is a complex experience and involves both sensory and emotional components at different order of neurons from the peripheral to the central nervous system. Once the painful impulse has been initiated and received by the brain, the interpretation of pain itself is based on interrelated biological, psychological, and social factors. That is why the sensation of pain is defined as "an unpleasant sensory and emotional experience associated with actual or potential tissue damage or described in terms of such damage" (Merskey et al. 1994).

Furthermore, pain can be modulated by the past experiences, emotions and cultural background of the person via sensory-discriminative, cognitive-behavioral and affective-emotional mechanisms. The transmission of pain information from the periphery to the cortex is therefore critically dependent upon integration and signal processing at the three levels of neurons within the CNS.

Clinically, a uni-dimensional measure using a numerical rating pain scale is commonly used, because of its convenience and reliability, to measure the intensity of neck pain. However, it cannot describe the whole range of the pain experience and the presence and severity of pain represents only a small part of the health outcome, especially in chronic pain syndrome.

THE EFFICACY OF THE TRADITIONAL DISEASE MODEL FOR MANAGEMENT OF NECK PAIN

The development of western medicine has a long history. The traditional Cartesian model of specific pain pathways (Foster 1901) is deeply rooted in the concepts of the clinical management of patients suffering from pain or disease. Pain is directly caused by tissue damage and the amount of pain is directly proportional to the extent of tissue damage. Tissue damage will cause impairments which in turn result in disability and/or inability to work. If we can treat the pain, the disability will also recover and patients will return to work.

Therefore, the common conservative management includes rest and pain killers, often prescribed by many medical practitioners in order to prevent further tissue damage. Various forms of physiotherapy include electrotherapy, traction, acupuncture, mobilization and massage prescribed by physiotherapists in order to promote tissue healing (Aker et al. 1996).

This traditional disease concept seems to work well for patients who have a clear-cut pathology identified and a positive attitude confronting the pain. However, this traditional management for patients with neck pain, from an evidence-based perspective, is now a point of controversy in the literature.

The use of medications was the most common practice for general practitioners in dealing with a patient's pain. Nevertheless, their effect on chronic neck pain was not promising in the literature. Oral psychotropic agents and cyclobenzaprine had been found to be in conflict in their effect on pain reduction (Peloso et al. 2005). Only limited evidence supported the usage of Non-Steroidal Anti-Inflammatory Drugs (NSAIDs) while the effect of eperison hydrochloride and tetrazepam stayed unclear as only one trial showed a positive result (Peloso et al. 2005).

For the physical modalities, TENS, laser therapy and therapeutic ultrasound, limited evidence has suggested they are ineffective in reducing neck pain (Aker et al. 1996 and Philadelphia panel 2001). Similarly, the evidence for the immediate reduction of pain after using a pulsed electromagnetic field is limited (Aker et al. 1996), and its long term effect is as yet unclear (Kroeling and Gross 2005). Graham et al. (2006) found that evidence supporting intermittent neck traction for pain reduction did exist in the literature, but it was limited and inconclusive. Similar evidence was found to not support continuous traction (Graham et al. 2006). Massage therapy, seemed to be an effective treatment, but its effect is still unclear because of the heterogeneity of the studies (Haraldsson et al. 2006). A non-significant benefit of using mobilization or manipulation alone in treating chronic neck pain has been shown in the literature (Ernst et al. 2006 and Gross et al. 2004).

Although there was clinical evidence that supported the efficacy of muscular strengthening in neck rehabilitation programmes (Highland et al. 1992 and Jordan et al. 1998), the effect of strengthening and stretching exercises on chronic mechanical neck disorders has been shown to be unclear in recent literature (Kay et al. 2005 and Sarig-Bahat 2003). Only minimal evidence supported stabilization exercise as an effective modality in dealing with chronic neck pain (Moffett et al. 2006). Even though there was limited evidence supporting the use of manipulation, mobilization or exercises alone, there was strong evidence of the benefit in combining the two as a treatment regime (Gross et al. 2004 and Kay et al. 2005).

With the advances in neurophysiology of pain and more research to investigate the relationship between pain, impairment, disability and incapacity for work, we know that the pure biomechanical causal model that "tissue damage causes pain" alone is inadequate to explain the different clinical presentations. This is especially true in chronic pain patients, as we cannot identify any structural damage and, in fact, pain is not the same as tissue damage: pain, impairment, disability and incapacity for work are weakly related (Waddell 2002).

On the contrary, a new trend in considering psychosocial factors in the management of spinal pain had been established (Linton et al. 2000 and Jensen et al. 1995). Evidence has shown that cognitive-behavioural interventions could be successful in preventing acute or subacute spinal problems from changing into chronic disability (Linton et al. 2000). There is also increasing evidence to show that the biopsychosocial model of human illness (rather than the pain or disease model), which consists of factors like attitudes and beliefs, coping strategies, illness behaviors, occupational demands and cultural attitudes may help to give a better understanding of management strategies for patients with chronic pain (Waddell 2004).

However, unlike lower back pain (European Commission 2004 and Guzman et al. 2001), this kind of intervention was still untried in its application to patients with neck pain (Karjalainen et al. 2003). More studies are required to build up sufficient evidence before it can be concluded that it is an effective intervention.

THE BIOPSYCHOSOCIAL MODEL

There is increasing evidence to support the belief that the clinical presentation of chronic disability could be better understood and managed by using a biopsychosocial model which, as its name implies, considers the influence and interaction of physical, psychological and social factors on human pain perception and behaviors (Waddell 2004).

Unlike the traditional Cartesian model of specific pain pathways (Foster 1901), the biopsychosocial model regards human chronic disability and pain as a human illness, rather than as a disease.

In this regard, although neck pain is a physical problem and arises from the nociceptors of the structures within the neck, its clinical presentation and its response to rehabilitation also depends on personal beliefs, lifestyle and social and physical environment, rather than biological function or medical care alone (Waddell 2004). Chronic disability is an equilibrium status resulting from an evolving and dynamic interaction between physical (e.g. tissue damage and physiological dysfunction) psychological (e.g. illness behavior, expectation, beliefs, emotion and distress) and social (e.g. culture, social interactions and sick role) elements over time. There is no clear-cut division between these three elements.

In terms of clinical management, instead of focusing on how to find out the physiological mechanisms of the disability, Waddell (2004) suggested that interventions should emphasize on the effects of interactions between the whole individual and the perceived environment. It is necessary to distinguish the underlying physical problem from the patient's reaction and illness behavior.

Apart from directing physical treatment to the physical problem according to the type and degree of tissue damage, it is important to address patients' hopes and fears, how they react and cope and behave. On the other hand, it is also important to consider how medical information and advice and the whole management process affect patients' beliefs and feelings and behavior.

It is essential to recognize and try to change mistaken beliefs and fears at an early stage to prevent chronicity. It is critical to keep in mind that the ultimate goal and outcome of health care is not only to relieve, or at least control, pain but also to help patients get on with their normal lives (Waddell 2004).

It is important to note that the interaction effects between these factors over time are very different at the acute, subacute and chronic stages. Each phase may involve a different set of interactions and the interactions might produce new properties, characteristics and effects. The biopsychosocial system cannot be reduced to the sum of its parts (Glouberman 2001). Therefore, timing and the appropriate kind of intervention strategy are critical factors in the psychosocial model.

THE FEAR-AVOIDANCE BELIEFS MODEL

Among the psychosocial factors, the fear-avoidance beliefs as set out in the Fear-Avoidance Beliefs Model developed by Lethem et al. (1983) have been hypothesized as one of the most important, specific and powerful cognitive variables in predicting disability and treatment outcome in patients with lower back pain (Crombez et al. 1999; Fritz et al. 2001; Vlaeyen et al. 1999).

The main basis of this model is the perception that pain is not only influenced by organic pathology but also by induced pain-related fears. Patients may react to these pain-related fears with avoidance behaviors like resting, antalgic posture, a limping gait, the use of supportive aids or by avoiding painful movements in order to reduce pain, promote healing and prevent re-injury.

However, persistent avoidance behaviors beyond the expected tissue-healing time will prolong and exaggerate the pain and fear, causing detrimental effects to patients both physically and psychosocially. It may at first seem that fear-avoidance beliefs are natural and accurate interpretations of pain as a signal of injury, but that is only part of the story. By the time pain becomes chronic, there is very little relation between fear-avoidance beliefs and pain itself, and fear of pain may be more disabling than pain itself.

In fact, these long-lasting fear-avoidance beliefs may lead to patients being unable to perform certain movements and activities of daily living and work because they anticipate that these movements and activities will increase pain even in the absence of tissue damage or that they will stop movements or activities because they overestimate their exertion rather than because of the increased pain.

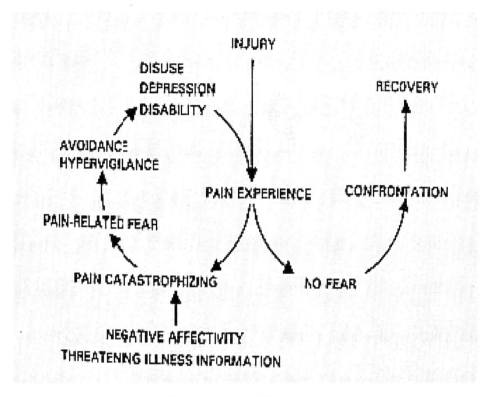

Figure 2. The Fear-Avoidance Model (Lethem et al. 1983).

In other words, patients develop or learn prejudgments based on past painful experiences and events and tend to relate to new situations that appear similar in a defensive way. Such beliefs therefore, are more disabling than the actual pain itself, and can thus subsequently cause disuse atrophy syndrome and may also lead to adaptative withdrawal from social activities and adaptation to a non-working situation. All those beliefs make it more difficult for the patient to return to normal living and work (Figure 2).

THE NEURO-MECHANISM PERSPECTIVES OF THE FEAR-AVOIDANCE BELIEFS MODEL

The main challenge for neuroscience researchers is to determine how the human central nervous system (CNS) controls motor behaviors. The CNS attracts multidisciplinary neuroscience researchers like physiologists, anatomists, pharmacologists, therapists, bioengineers and psychologists, who try to approach this question with different experimental designs, varying from molecular and electrophysiological to cognitive and behavioral perspectives and from non-vertebrae to vertebrae and primate species.

One of the main focuses of this central neuroscience question for the modern neuroscientist is to understand how the feedforward and feedback mechanisms operate within the CNS to produce simple motor movements such as locomotion and to maintain postural control in reaction to stimuli from the external environment.

The advances in neuro-imaging techniques, have led to the development of functional Magnetic Resonance Imaging (fMRI), an imaging technique sensitive to changes in regional blood oxygenation as an index of neuronal activity, which has been used with wide success in the mapping of human brain functions and in characterizing the CNS pathways (Cohen and Bookheimer 1994).

Another advanced neuro-imaging technique is the Positron Emission Tomography (PET) which involves the acquisition of physiologic images based on the detection of radiation from the emission of positrons administered to the body. It studies the physiological processes involved in metabolically active molecules within the brain.

With these advanced neuro-imaging techniques, we now have a better understanding of how seemingly simple pain responses are executed. Neuroscientists can now analyze the relationship of differential activation pattern of brain regions to particular dimensions of pain, and they can also start to disentangle subprocesses within the nociceptive system by characterizing the role of individual regions within the brain with different stimulus intensities (Bornhövd et al. 2002).

Based on the abundance of neuroscience research data available, the common finding is that while somatosensory cortical area activity is closely associated with the coding of pain intensity, the rostral part of the anterior cingulate cortex (ACC), which has extensive connections to the amygdala and periaqueductal gray matter, is a key modulator of the internal emotional response to pain. It is critical in establishing fear-avoidance pain-response behaviors (Devinsky et al. 1995; Davis and Whalen 2001; Bornhövd et al. 2002; Gao et al. 2004).

Amygdalae are an almond-shaped group of nuclei located deep in the hippocampus and the temporal horn of the lateral ventricle of the brain. The amygdala is divided into three groups of subnuclei, the large basolateral, the smaller corticomedial and the central groups. It receives sensory input from widespread areas of the nervous system including somatosensory, visual, auditory and visceral stimuli and its key role is the control of the autonomic nervous system function.

The mode of amygdale control of autonomic nervous system function differs from that of the hypothalamus. The hypothalamus's control of the autonomic nervous system function is reflex in nature via baroreceptors and osmoreceptors whereas control of autonomic nervous system activity by the amygdala is mediated by previous experiences (Patestas and Gartner 2006).

Furthermore, the evidence that anticipation of pain itself could trigger top-down mechanisms in modulating cortical nociceptive systems even in the absence of actual noxious input, suggests that the activity of cortical nociceptive networks may be directly influenced by cognitive factors (Porro et al. 2002).

In an animal behavior study, monkeys with bilateral removal of the amygdala showed marked changes in emotional behavior (Davis et al. 2002). They would exhibit behavior involving loss of fear inhibition, such as approaching objects without hesitation and examining objects by mouth, rather than with their hands. Excitotoxic lesion of amygdala and ACC in rats will result in loss of fear inhibition behaviors in response to noxious stimulus. (Gao et al. 2004).

Moreover, Lei et al. (2004) found that in rats with fear-avoidance behaviors, significantly higher levels of Fos expression (as a marker of neuronal activity) can be observed in particular areas, including ACC and amygdala. In human, activations in the amygdala during noxious stimulus have been reported (Derbyshire et al. 1997; Bornhövd et al. 2002). However, movement is not permitted during imaging studies, therefore, it will be much more difficult to investigate using imaging techniques which part of the brain(s) is/are essentially activated to movements during the effect of pain-related fear.

Although both electrophysiological and animal behavior studies provided considerable evidence that the anterior cingulated cortex and the amygdala are particular brain regions that may be the basis of fear- avoidance and its associated behavioral changes, one should notice that signals processing in the central network of the nociceptive system are both in parallel and in series with other brain regions. That means other brain regions which may not primarily subserve the basis of fear-avoidance behavior, still exert their effect in it.

It should be emphasized that cognitive feedback is an essential factor and it is constantly being monitored in the central nervous system in order to carry out the motor performance efficiently and accurately, and updates are being operated as a consequence of new experiences.

Moreover, pain itself does not always produce fear. Sportsmen or soldiers, for example, might accept pain as a normal part of training. Fear, on the other hand, is a powerful negative drive in humans and animals, closely allied to pain. Fear is to some extent an inborn instinct, but to a greater extent it is learned.

Therefore, the exact neuro-mechanisms of pain-related fear and its associated avoidance behaviors are complex and remain largely uncertain.

THE FEAR-AVOIDANCE BELIEFS QUESTIONNAIRE

Waddell et al. (1993) developed the Fear-Avoidance Beliefs Questionnaire (FABQ) in order to measure fear-avoidance beliefs in patients with lower back pain. It is a 16-item, self-reporting questionnaire, in which each item is graded on a 7-point Likert scale ('strongly disagree' to 'strongly agree'). It has two subscales shown by factor analysis, one subscale focusing on patients' beliefs about how physical activities affect their pain (FABQ_PA) and the other focusing on patients' beliefs about how work affects their pain (FABQ_W). The FABQ score is calculated by adding up individual item scores. A higher total score indicates a higher level of fear-avoidance beliefs.

This questionnaire has proven reliability, validity and ability to predict treatment outcome and disability in patients with lower back pain (Waddell et al. 1993; Klenerman et al. 1995 and Pfingsten et al. 1997).

Apart from FABQ, there are also two other reliable measurements, the Tampa Scale of Kinesiophobia, (TSK) (Kori et al. 1990) and the Pain Catastrophizing Scale, (PCS) (Sullivan et al. 1995) developed to assess and quantify the constructs of fear-avoidance beliefs.

Both the 17-item TSK and the 16-item FABQ are valid questionnaires with good internal consistency and substantial test–retest reliability. However, the TSK is aimed more at measuring a fear of (re)injury, whereas the FABQ measures more a fear of pain directly caused by physical activities and work. That may explain why the concurrent validity between TSK and FABQ (physical activity subscale) is 'moderately strong' to 'strong', and higher than between TSK and FABQ (work subscale) (Swinkels-Meewisse et al. 2003).

The Pain Catastrophizing Scale has 13 items which divide into 3 subscales: rumination, magnification and helplessness. It has moderate correlations among the three subscales (r = 0.6 to 0.87) and high internal consistency (r = 0.87) (Sullivan et al. 1995). It was developed to measure exaggerated negative focus on pain sensations and was found to have a significant correlation with depression, anxiety and fear of pain. However, it does not have any work-related content in the questionnaire, which is important for patients with work-related chronic pain.

PSYCHOMETRIC PROPERTIES OF THE FEAR-AVOIDANCE BELIEFS QUESTIONNAIRE IN PATIENTS WITH NECK PAIN

The present authors conducted an observational corss-sectional and prospective study to investigate the validity and reliability of the Chinese version of the Fear-avoidance Beliefs Questionnaire in patients with neck pain. (Lee et al. 2006) Four samples with 476 consecutive adult patients with neck pain were recruited from four physiotherapy centers. The original questionnaire was translated into Chinese by forward and backward translation and reviewed by expert panels. (Appendix I and II) The subjects completed the Chinese version of the fear-avoidance questionnaire, Northwick Park Neck Pain Questionnaire, Medical Outcomes 36-Item Short-Form Health Survey and their pain intensity was measured using the 11-point pain numerical rating scale.

They were observed and measured at the beginning of physiotherapy, at week 3 and at week 6 after treatment began. Results demonstrated that the questionnaire had very good content validity and test-retest reliability with an intraclass correlation coefficient of 0.81 and the Cronbach's alpha coefficient of 0.90.

Spearman's correlation coefficients between fear-avoidance and the neck pain questionnaire, the health survey (Physical), health survey (Mental) and pain scale were 0.56, 0.45, 0.36 and 0.34 respectively. The standard response mean and effect size at week six after treatment begun was 0.38 and 0.32 respectively.

Factor analysis yielded three factors which accounted for 61.6% of the total variance of the questionnaire and is interestingly consistent with the finding in the study of the German version of fear-avoidance questionnaire in patients with lower back pain (Pfingsten et al. 2000).

This gives good support to conclude that the Fear-avoidance Beliefs Questionnaire is a valid and reliable tool for patients with neck pain. It has been shown to demonstrate very good content validity, a high degree of test-retest reliability and internal consistency, good construct validity and medium responsiveness.

THE ROLE OF FEAR-AVOIDANCE BELIEFS IN PATIENTS WITH NECK PAIN: RELATIONSHIPS WITH CURRENT AND FUTURE DISABILITY AND WORK CAPACITY

Although neck pain is believed to be of multifactorial origin, there is increasing evidence that both physical and psychosocial risk factors can contribute to its development, and cultural and psychosocial factors are more important predictors of chronicity of neck pain, prolonged work loss and restricted work capacity (Croft et al. 2001 and Trinkoff et al. 2002). Previous studies showed that the fear-avoidance model is not limited to lower back pain patients but it is present in a wide range of patients with chronic pain conditions (Rose et al. 1992). A study of patients with neck pain and patients with back pain has revealed that fear-avoidance beliefs are present in both (George et al. 2001). The present authors have found that the construct of fear-avoidance beliefs can also be applied to patients with neck pain. (Lee et al. 2006)

In a recent prospective observational study the present authors investigated the relationship between the fear-avoidance beliefs and future disability and work capacity in patients with neck pain. (Lee et al. 2007) A total of 120 subjects with a diagnosis of neck pain and an incomplete work status were recruited from the physiotherapy out-patient clinics of two major hospitals in Hong Kong.

Subjects underwent examination of the active neck range of movements and neck muscle strength and completed the Fear-avoidance Beliefs Questionnaire, the Northwick Park Neck Pain Questionnaire, the Medical Outcomes 36-Item Short-Form Health Survey and the 11-point pain numerical rating scale. These were assessed at the beginning and week 6 of the rehabilitation programs. Subjects' work capacity was assessed at week 6 and 3 months after the 6-week rehabilitation programs. Subjects were assigned into the 6-week conventional physiotherapy or the individualized exercise training scheduled for 2 therapy sessions per week for 6 weeks.

Results of the study showed that all the Fear-Avoidance Beliefs Questionnaire subscales were moderately correlated with initial pain, disability and health measure scores but had a low correlation with neck active range of movement index and not significantly correlated with neck muscle strength index and age. (However, the Spearman's correlation coefficients between fear-avoidance beliefs and initial and week 6 disability levels were 0.47 and 0.48 respectively.) Regression analysis showed that the fear-avoidance beliefs significantly improved the goodness of fit of the model for predicting week 6 disability levels and return to complete work capacity at week 6 and 3 months after the rehabilitation program even after controlling for the physical impairments, the health status, the pain intensity, the initial disability level and the type of treatment received.

The results of the present study may provide evidence to show the unique characteristic or construct of the cognitive influence of fear-avoidance beliefs from other measures and give further evidence to support the theory that fear-avoidance beliefs factor was an important variable in predicting future disability and return to complete work capacity in patients with neck pain at the earlier phase of rehabilitation.

Since prolonged work incapacity played an important role in socioeconomic impacts, early identification of patients at risk of prolonged work incapacity was essential in order to implement appropriate interventions targeted to this subgroup of patients.

Therefore, fear-avoidance beliefs factor should be considered in the management of neck pain in the initial stage of rehabilitation.

APPENDIX I. THE CHINESE VERSION OF FEAR-AVOIDANCE BELIEF QUESTIONNAIRE

頸痛恐懼逃避信念問卷

以下是其他病人告訴我們的一些關於他們的痛楚的事情。請為每一句子圈出任何由0至6的數字，以表示各種體力活動，如閱讀、攜帶物件、走路、開車等，影響或會影響您頸部痛楚的程度。

	完全不同意			不肯定			完全同意
1. 我的痛楚是由體力活動所導致	0	1	2	3	4	5	6
2. 體力活動會使我的痛楚加劇	0	1	2	3	4	5	6
3. 體力活動可能會弄傷我的頸部	0	1	2	3	4	5	6
4. 我不應該進行使(或可能使)我痛楚加劇的體力活動	0	1	2	3	4	5	6
5. 我不能夠進行使(或可能使)我痛楚加劇的體力活動	0	1	2	3	4	5	6

以下的句子是關於您的正常工作如何影響或會影響您的頸部痛楚。

	完全不同意			不肯定			完全同意
6. 我的痛楚是由我的工作或工作時的意外所導致	0	1	2	3	4	5	6
7. 我的工作觸發我的痛楚	0	1	2	3	4	5	6
8. 我會為我的痛楚索取賠償	0	1	2	3	4	5	6
9. 我的工作量對我來說太多了	0	1	2	3	4	5	6
10. 我的工作使我或會使我的痛楚加劇	0	1	2	3	4	5	6
11. 我的工作可能會弄傷我的頸部	0	1	2	3	4	5	6
12. 以我現時的痛楚，我不應該進行我的正常工作	0	1	2	3	4	5	6
13. 以我現時的痛楚，我不能夠進行我的正常工作	0	1	2	3	4	5	6
14. 未醫好痛楚之前，我不能夠進行我的正常工作	0	1	2	3	4	5	6
15. 我不認為在三個月內我會回到我的正常工作崗位	0	1	2	3	4	5	6
16. 我不認為我能夠再做那份工作	0	1	2	3	4	5	6

APPENDIX II. THE ENGLISH VERSION OF FEAR-AVOIDANCE BELIEF QUESTIONNAIRE

Fear-Avoidance Beliefs Questionnaire

Here are some of the things which other patients have told us about their pain. For each statement please circle any number from 0 to 6 to say how much physical activities such as reading, carrying, walking or driving affect or would affect your neck pain.

	Completely disagree			Unsure			Completely agree
1. My pain was caused by physical activities	0	1	2	3	4	5	6
2. Physical activity makes my pain worse	0	1	2	3	4	5	6
3. Physical activity might harm my neck	0	1	2	3	4	5	6
4. I should not do physical activities which (might) make my pain worse	0	1	2	3	4	5	6
5. I cannot do physical activities which (might) make my pain worse	0	1	2	3	4	5	6

The following statements are about how your normal work affects or would affect your neck pain.

	Completely disagree			Unsure			Completely agree
6. My pain was caused by my work or by an accident at work	0	1	2	3	4	5	6
7. My work aggravated my pain	0	1	2	3	4	5	6
8. I have a claim for compensation for my pain	0	1	2	3	4	5	6
9. My work is too heavy for me	0	1	2	3	4	5	6
10. My work makes or would make my pain worse	0	1	2	3	4	5	6
11. My work might harm my neck	0	1	2	3	4	5	6
12. I should not do my normal work with my present pain	0	1	2	3	4	5	6
13. I cannot do my normal work with my present pain	0	1	2	3	4	5	6
14. I cannot do my normal work till my pain is treated	0	1	2	3	4	5	6
15. I do not think that I will be back to my normal work within 3 months	0	1	2	3	4	5	6
16. I do not think that I will eve be able to go back to that work	0	1	2	3	4	5	6

REFERENCES

Aker PD, Gross AR, Goldsmith CH and Peloso P. Conservative management of mechanical neck pain: systemic overview and meta-analysis. *British Medical Journal*. 1996; 313: 1291 - 1296.

Bolay H and Moskowitz MA. Mechanisms of pain modulation in chronic syndromes. *Neurology*. 2002; 59: S2 - 7.

Borghouts JA, Koes BW, Vondeling H, and Bouter LM. Cost-of-illness of neck pain in the Netherlands in 1996. *Pain*. 1999;80:629-636.

Bornhövd K, Quante M, Glauche V, Bromm B, Weiller C and Büchel C. Painful stimuli evoke different stimulus–response functions in the amygdala, prefrontal, insula and somatosensory cortex: a single-trial fMRI study. *Brain*. 2002; 125: 1326 - 1336.

Cohen MS and Bookheimer SY. Localization of brain function using magnetic resonance imaging. *Trends in Neurosciences*. 1994; 17: 268 - 277.

Croft PR, Lewis M, Papageorgiou AC, Thomas E, Jayson MIV, Macfarlane GJ and Silman AJ. Risk factors for neck pain: a longitudinal study in the general population. *Pain*. 2001; 93: 317 - 325.

Crombez G, Vlaeyen JWS, Heuts PH and Lysens R. Pain-related fear is more disabling than pain itself: evidence on the role of pain-related fear in chronic back pain disability. *Pain*. 1999; 80: 329 - 340.

Davis M and Whalen PJ. The amygdale: vililance and emotion. *Molecular Psychiatry*. 2001; 6: 13 - 34.

Derbyshire SWG, Jones AKP, Gyulai F, Clark S, Townsend D and Firestone LL. Pain processing during three level of noxious stimulation produces differential patterns of central activity. *Pain.* 1997; 73: 431-445.

Devinsky O, Morrell MJ and Vogt BA. Contributions of anterior cingulate cortex to behavior. *Brain.* 1995; 118: 279 - 306.

Ernst E and Canter PH. A systematic review of systematic reviews of spinal manipulation. *Journal of the Royal Society of Medicine.* 2006; 99(4): 192 - 196.

European Commission. European guidelines for the management of chronic low back pain. Research Directorate General, European Commission. 2004. COST Action B13. Available at: www.backpaineurope.org.

Fejer R, Kyvik KO and Hartvigsen J. The prevalence of neck pain in the world population: a systematic critical review of the literature. *Eur. Spin. J.* 2006; 15(6):834-848.

Foster M. Lectures on the history of physiology during the sixteenth, seventeenth and eighteenth centuries. Cambridge: Cambridge University Press, 1901.

Fritz JM, George SZ and Delitto A. The role of fear-avoidance beliefs in acute low back pain:relationships with current and future disability and work status. *Pain.* 2001; 94: 7 – 15.

Gao YJ, Ren WH, Zhang YQ and Zhao ZQ. Contributions of the anterior cingulated cortex and amygdale to pain- and fear-conditioned place avoidance in rats. *Pain.* 2004; 110: 343 - 353.

George SZ, Fritz JM and Erhard RE. A comparison of fear-avoidance beliefs in patients with lumbar spine pain and cervical spine pain. *Spine.* 2001; 26: 2139 - 2145.

Glouberman S. Towards a new perspective on health policy. Canadian policy research networks study. 2001. Available online at: http//www.cprn.org/cprn.htm 2001.

Graham N. Gross AR. Goldsmith C and Cervical Overview Group. Mechanical traction for mechanical neck disorders: a systematic review. *Journal of Rehabilitation Medicine.* 2006; 38(3):145 – 152.

Gross AR, Hoving JL, Haines TA, Goldsmith CH, Kay T, Aker P, Bronfort G and Cervical Overview Group. Manipulation and mobilisation for mechanical neck disorders. *Cochrane Database of Systematic Reviews.* 2004; 1: CD004249.

Guzman J, Esmail R, Karjalainen K, Malmivaara, Irvin E and Bombardier C. Multidisciplinary rehabilitation for chronic low back pain: systematic review. *British Medical Journal.* 2001; 322: 1511 - 1516.

Haraldsson BG, Gross AR, Myers CD, Ezzo JM, Morien A, Goldsmith C, Peloso PM, Bronfort G and Cervical Overview Group. Massage for mechanical neck disorders. *Cochrane Database of Systematic Reviews.* 2006; 3: CD004871.

Highland TR, Dresisinger TE, Laura LV, Russell GS. Changes in isometric strength and range of motion of the isolated cervical spine after eight weeks of clinical rehabilitation. *Spine.* 1992; 17 (6 suppl): S77 - 82.

Jensen I, Nygren A and Gamberale F. The role of the psychologist in multidisciplinary treatments for chronic neck and shoulder pain: a controlled cost-effectiveness study. *Scandinavian Journal of Rehabilitation Medicine.* 1995; 27(1): 19 - 26.

Jordan A, Bendix T, Nielsen H, Hansen FR, Høst D and Winkel A. Intensive training, physiotherapy, or manipulation for patients with chronic neck pain: a prospective, single-blinded, randomized clinical trial. *Spine.* 1998; 23(3): 311 - 319.

Karjalainen K, Malmivaara A, van Tulder M, Roine R, Jauhiainen M, Hurri H and Koes BW. Multidisciplinary biopsychosocial rehabilitation for neck and shoulder pain among working age adults. *Cochrane Database of Systematic Reviews*. 2003; 2: CD002194.

Kay TM, Gross A, Goldsmith C, Santaguida PL, Hoving J, Bronfort G and Cervical Overview Group. Exercises for mechanical neck disorders. *Cochrane Database of Systematic Reviews*. 2005; 3: CD004250.

Klenerman L, Slade PD, Stanley IM, Pennie B, Reilly JP, Atchinson LE, Troup JD and Rose MJ. The prediction of chronicity in patients with an acute attack of low back pain in a general practice setting. *Spine*. 1995; 20: 478 - 484.

Kori SH, Miller RP and Todd DD. Kinesophobia: A new view of chronic pain behaviour. *Pain Management*. 1990:35–43.

Kroeling P, Gross A, Houghton PE and Cervical Overview Group. Electrotherapy for neck disorders (Review). *Cochrane Database of Systematic Reviews*. 2005; 2: CD004251.

Lee KC, Chiu TW, Lam TH. Psychometric Properties of the Fear-avoidance Beliefs Questionnaire in Patients with Neck Pain. *Clinical Rehabilitation* 2006; 20: 909-920.

Lee KC, Chiu TW, Lam TH. The role of fear-avoidance beliefs in patients with neck pain: relationships with current and future disability and work capacity. *Clinical Rehabilitation* 2007; 21:812-821.

Lei LG, Zhang YQ and Zhao ZQ. Pain-related aversion and Fos expression in the central nervous system in rats. *Neuroreport*. 2004; 15(1): 67-71.

Lethem J, Slade PD, Troup JDG and Bentley G. Outline of a fear-avoidance model of exaggerated pain perceptions. *Behaviour Research and Therapy*. 1983; 21: 401 - 408.

Linton SJ and Andersson T. Can chronic disability be prevented? A randomized trail of a cognitive-behavior intervention and two forms of information for patients with spinal problems. *Spine*. 2000; 25: 2825 - 2831.

Merskey H and Bogduk N, eds. Classification of chronic pain: descriptions of chronic pain syndromes and definitions of pain terms. Seattle: IASP Press, 1994, 2nd ed. p103 - 111.

Moffett J and McLean S. The role of physiotherapy in the management of non-specific back pain and neck pain. *Rheumatology*. 2006; 45(4): 371 - 378.

Patestas MA and Gartner LP. A textbook of neuroanatomy. Maden MA: Blackwell Science Ltd 2006.

Peloso P, Gross A, Haines T, Trinh K, Goldsmith CH, Aker P and Cervical Overview Group. Medicinal and injection therapies for mechanical neck disorders. *Cochrane Database of Systematic Reviews*. 2005; 2: CD000319.

Pfingsten M, Leibing E, Franz C, Franz C and Saur P. Effectiveness of a multimodal treatment program for chronic low-back pain. *Pain*. 1997; 73: 77 - 85.

Pfingsten M, Kroner-Herwig B, Leibing E, Kronshage U and Hildebrandt J. Validation of the German version of the fear-avoidance beliefs questionnaire (FABQ). *European Journal of Pain*. 2000; 4: 259 - 266.

Philadelphia Panel. Evidence-based clinical practice guidelines on selected rehabilitation interventions for neck pain. *Physical Therapy*. 2001; 81: 1701 - 1717.

Porro CA, Baraldi P, Pagnoni G, Serafini M, Facchin P, Maieron M and Nichelli P. Does anticipation of pain affect cortical nociceptive systems? *Journal of Neuroscience*. 2002; 22(8): 3206 - 3214.

Rose MJ, Klenerman L, Atchison L and Slade PD. An application of the fear avoidance model to three chronic pain problems. *Behaviour Research and Therapy*. 1992; 30: 359 - 365.

Sarig-Bahat H. Evidence for exercise therapy in mechanical neck disorders. *Manual Therapy*. 2003; 8: 10 - 20.

Sullivan, MJL, Bishop SR and Pivik J. The Pain Catastrophizing Scale: development and validation. *Psychological Assessment*. 1995; 7(4): 524 - 532.

Swinkels-Meewisse EJ, Swinkels RA, Verbeek AL, Vlaeyen JW and Oostendorp RA. Psychometric properties of the Tampa Scale for kinesiophobia and the fear-avoidance beliefs questionnaire in acute low back pain. *Manual Therapy*. 2003; 8(1): 29 - 36.

Trinkoff AM, Lipscomb JA, Geiger-Brown J, and Brady B. Musculoskeletal problems of the neck, shoulder, and back and functional consequences in nurses. *Am. J. Ind. Med.* 2002;41:170–8.

Vlaeyen JWS, Seelen HAM, Peters M, De Jong P, Aretz E, Beisiegel E and Weber WE. Fear of movement / (re)injury and muscular reactivity in chronic low back pain patients: an experimental investigation. *Pain*. 1999; 82: 297 - 304.

Waddell G. Models of disability: using low back pain as an example. London: Royal Society of Medicine Press, 2002.

Waddell G. The back pain revolution. Edinburgh: *Churchill Livingstone*, 2004, 2nd ed.

Waddell G, Newton M, Henderson I, Somerville D and Main CJ. A fear avoidance beliefs questionnaire (FABQ) and the role of fear-avoidance beliefs in chronic low back pain and disability. *Pain*. 1993; 52: 157 - 168.

INDEX

A

abuse, 86, 104, 118
access, 50
accounting, 103
acetaminophen, x, 69, 82, 83, 84, 119, 121, 135, 142
acetylcholine, 89, 95, 98, 133
acid, 71, 72, 74, 75, 76, 78, 79, 80, 81, 82, 92, 100, 109, 110, 111, 112, 113, 120, 137, 139, 140, 141
acidity, 79
action potential, 79
active compound, 111, 137
acupuncture, 34, 104, 105, 108, 109, 114, 123, 124, 126, 133, 141, 146
adalimumab, 93
adaptation, 34, 35, 149
adenosine, 72, 79, 94, 110, 116, 117, 129, 131, 134, 138
adhesions, 36
adolescents, 10
adults, vii, ix, 2, 10, 11, 41, 52, 55, 57, 58, 59, 64, 70, 120, 134, 157
advancement, 52
adverse effects, 97
adverse event, 110
afferent nerve, 75
age, ix, xi, 21, 33, 38, 52, 54, 58, 59, 70, 85, 102, 114, 116, 144, 153, 157
aggregation, 84, 99
aggression, 121
agonist, 85, 88, 90, 92, 94, 100, 101, 122, 133, 138
AIDS, 138
alcohol, 107
alcoholism, 104
allergic reaction, 97, 100
allergy, 97, 108
alternative medicine, 104
alters, 37, 38, 81, 140
amino, 9, 72, 74, 75, 100, 109, 139, 141

amino acid, 9, 72, 74, 75, 139, 141
amphibians, 74
amplitude, 59, 61
amygdala, 144, 150, 151, 155
anaerobe, 51
anaerobic bacteria, 48, 54, 102, 118
analgesic, 73, 76, 80, 82, 83, 84, 85, 86, 90, 91, 92, 93, 95, 96, 97, 98, 100, 104, 106, 110, 111, 112, 113, 118, 119, 121, 126, 129, 132, 133, 134, 135, 136, 139, 140, 141
anatomic site, 86
anatomy, 3, 12, 36, 38, 40, 42
anesthetics, x, 69, 100
aneurysm, 46
angina, 52, 54, 55
animal behavior, 150, 151
ankles, 75
ankylosing spondylitis, 93, 118
ANOVA, viii, ix, 17, 20, 28, 29, 30, 33
anterior cingulate cortex, 145, 150, 156
anterior cruciate, 122
antibiotic, 46, 51, 52, 53, 56, 103, 137
antibody, 90, 122
anticoagulation, 53
anticonvulsant, 92
antidepressant, 93, 96
antidepressants, 92, 93, 136
antigenicity, 89
antimicrobial therapy, 102, 136
antioxidant, 113
antipyretic, 83, 84, 111, 112, 119
anxiety, 36, 37, 42, 145, 152
aorta, 80
appetite, 95
apples, 113
arachnoiditis, 131
arrest, 99
artery, 46, 47, 86, 97, 99, 117, 118

arthritis, 46, 73, 75, 79, 83, 87, 93, 94, 95, 98, 106, 107, 109, 110, 112, 113, 115, 116, 121, 123, 125, 129, 135, 140
arthroplasty, 130
arthroscopy, 85, 122
articular cartilage, 2, 3, 117, 119
aspartate, 72, 91, 127, 128, 136, 140
aspartic acid, 141
aspiration, 50
assessment, x, 19, 32, 42, 58, 66, 113, 114, 118, 126
assignment, 116
asthma, 95
asymptomatic, ix, 57, 58, 59, 64, 90
ATP, 72, 75, 77, 81, 94, 110, 123, 130, 133
atrophy, 149
attitudes, 147
authors, xi, 113, 114, 143, 152, 153
autoimmune disease, 93
autoimmune diseases, 93
autonomic nervous system, 150
aversion, 157
avoidance, x, 143, 148, 150, 151, 152, 153, 154, 156, 157, 158
awareness, ix, 40, 45, 99
axon terminals, 100
axons, 8

B

bacillus, 88
back pain, x, 6, 34, 37, 70, 71, 85, 86, 90, 92, 93, 107, 108, 114, 116, 119, 120, 121, 124, 137, 140, 143, 147, 148, 151, 152, 153, 155, 156, 157, 158
background, x, 143, 145
bacteremia, 53
bacteria, 46, 49, 101, 102, 103, 118
base, 37, 47, 48
behavior, 73, 126, 129, 147, 148, 150, 151, 156, 157
behaviors, x, 86, 140, 143, 147, 148, 149, 150, 151
beliefs, x, 143, 147, 148, 149, 151, 153, 156, 157, 158
bending, 5
beneficial effect, x, 69, 92
benefits, 36, 38
benign, 102, 136
beverages, 110
binding, 84, 94, 100, 101, 129, 139
biochemistry, 34
biofeedback, 106
biological activity, 89, 94
biologically active compounds, 137
biomechanics, vii, 1, 3, 10, 13, 36
biosynthesis, 80, 110, 120

bipedal, ix, x, 57, 58, 65, 66
bladder, 87
bleeding, 97
blepharospasm, 89, 117, 133
blocks, 89, 94, 111, 119, 142
body weight, 59
bone, 2, 3, 6, 18, 35, 47, 70, 101, 102, 103, 106, 107, 124, 126, 128, 129, 130, 133, 136, 137
brachial plexus, 117, 124
bradycardia, 90
bradykinin, 72, 73, 77, 81, 85, 105, 119
brain, 74, 76, 77, 79, 85, 90, 92, 95, 100, 132, 135, 139, 144, 145, 150, 151, 155
breakdown, 110
bronchial asthma, 95
burn, 71
burning, 87, 96, 144

C

cadaver, 13
calcitonin, x, 3, 11, 12, 69, 72, 73, 74, 75, 116, 122, 132, 135, 138, 141, 144
calcium, 75, 76, 77, 87, 92, 95, 100, 106, 132, 134, 139, 141
caliber, 9
Canada, 135
cancer, 95, 96, 98, 100, 130, 134, 138, 140
candidates, 104
cannabinoids, 95, 141
capsule, vii, viii, 1, 2, 3, 5, 6, 7, 8, 9, 10, 11, 12, 14, 15
car accidents, 12
cardiac tamponade, 49
carpal tunnel syndrome, 30, 32
cartilage, 6, 18, 48, 94, 109, 110, 112, 117, 119
case studies, 96
catheter, 98
cation, 79, 140
causality, 58
causation, 18, 32
cefazolin, 101, 103, 104, 123, 130
cell, 77, 81, 94, 100, 107, 110, 111, 123
cell membranes, 110
cellulitis, 46, 48, 52, 53
central nervous system, vii, 1, 6, 8, 9, 11, 72, 73, 87, 91, 94, 104, 145, 149, 151, 157
cephalosporin, 51, 101, 103
cerebral palsy, 37, 42
cerebrospinal fluid, 77
certification, viii, 33
cervical radiculopathy, 119, 128
cervical spondylosis, 85, 105, 124

challenges, 32
channel blocker, 79, 92, 128
channels, 75, 79, 95, 100, 117
chemical, 36, 72, 78, 79, 81, 84, 111, 128
chemiluminescence, 119
chemokines, 79
chemotaxis, 78
childhood, 52
children, 41, 52, 54, 55, 56, 102, 118, 136, 141
China, 1, 12
choline, 138
cholinesterase, 95, 133
chondrocyte, 125
chondroitin sulfate, 109, 119
chromosome, 74, 80
circulation, 38, 83, 106
classes, 115
classification, 7, 91
clients, 37
cloning, 119
cluster headache, 88
clusters, 8
CNS, vii, 1, 9, 11, 40, 131, 146, 149, 150
coagulopathy, 97
coal, 32, 83
cocaine, 86, 137
coccyx, 48
coding, 150
cognitive variables, x, 143, 148
cohort, 106, 114, 118
collagen, 35, 36, 38, 39, 42, 107
collateral, 79
collateral damage, 79
combination therapy, 120
commercial, 93
common symptoms, 48
communication, 21, 39
communities, 34
community, 67
compatibility, 125
compensation, 31, 114, 125
complaints, 71, 118
complexity, 115, 145
compliance, 82, 127
complications, ix, 45, 46, 49, 50, 53, 97, 99, 140
components, 114, 122, 145
compounds, 79, 87, 106, 113
compression, vii, 1, 3, 4, 5, 6, 11, 14, 38, 51, 67, 100, 105, 109
computed tomography, 51, 54
computer, vii, viii, 6, 8, 17, 18, 19, 21, 22, 26, 30, 31, 32
computer use, vii, viii, 17, 18, 19, 22, 26, 30, 31, 32

concentration, 75, 81, 101, 137
conductance, 100
conduction, 75, 87, 88, 127
conflict, 146
connective tissue, 35, 36, 38, 39, 46, 48, 107, 112
constipation, 86
constituents, 137
construct validity, 152
consumption, 86
contour, 8, 35
controversial, 53, 86, 102
convergence, 40
cooling, 79, 94
coping strategies, 147
coping strategy, 114
correlation, 6, 9, 37, 38, 140, 152, 153
cortex, 145, 146, 150, 151, 155, 156
cortical bone, 101, 126
corticosteroids, 98, 99, 117
cost, viii, xi, 17, 19, 51, 144, 156
coupling, 79
covering, 53
critical analysis, 130
cross-sectional study, 31, 114
crying, 145
crystalline, 87, 88
culture, 51, 103, 147
curcumin, 137
cure, 103
cyclooxygenase, 83, 84, 111, 113, 119, 130
cytochrome, 83
cytokines, 9, 72, 73, 77, 78, 79, 81, 93, 112
cytotoxicity, 134

D

daily living, 34, 70, 148
damages, 84
danger, 47, 48
data analysis, 27
data collection, 18, 27
data gathering, 34
data set, ix, 34
debridement, 52, 53, 122
deficit, x, 66, 69, 99, 104
definition, 71
deformation, 3
degenerative conditions, 18
degradation, 94, 101, 122, 131
delivery, 95, 96, 125, 140
demographic structure, 19, 30
dependent variable, 60, 61
depression, 36, 105, 110, 114, 118, 133, 152

dermis, 39, 47, 83
destruction, 73, 75, 86
detection, 7, 71, 150
deviation, 51
diabetes, 25, 104
diabetic neuropathy, 88, 92, 96
diffusion, 90
direct action, 84
direct cost, viii, 17, 19
direct measure, 65
disability, x, 41, 70, 105, 113, 114, 118, 120, 121, 123, 125, 128, 143, 146, 147, 148, 151, 153, 155, 156, 157, 158
disaster, 55
discharges, 6
discitis, x, 69, 102, 103, 120
discomfort, vii, viii, 17, 18, 19, 24, 25, 27, 30, 31, 32, 39, 96, 105
discs, 3, 18, 77, 103, 127, 136
disease activity, 94, 110
disease model, 147
diseases, 48, 125, 128, 131
diskitis, 118, 136
disorder, 18, 25, 31, 46, 53, 88, 89, 100, 114
displacement, 4, 8, 53
dissociation, 132
distress, 52, 56, 147
distribution, 7, 21, 22, 35, 37, 38, 39, 42, 86
division, 147
docosahexaenoic acid, 79
dogs, 91, 129
dorsal horn, vii, 2, 10, 11, 15, 72, 73, 74, 75, 76, 81, 83, 91, 98, 122, 123, 127, 129, 132, 133, 134, 144
dosage, 106
dosing, 82
double blind study, 90
drainage, 46, 52
duration, 71, 92, 95, 100, 105, 106, 114, 117
dysphagia, 48, 52
dyspnea, 48
dystonia, 88, 89, 92, 101, 115, 117, 119, 120, 122, 133, 139, 140, 141

E

edema, 50, 51, 73
editors, 42, 132
education, 114, 125
effusion, 49
eicosapentaenoic acid, 79
elastin, 38
elbows, 24, 36
elderly, 105, 124, 135

elders, 67
electrodes, 14
emboli, 53, 99
embolization, 99
embolus, 49
EMG, 27
employees, 18
EMU, 21
encoding, 74, 116, 119
endorphins, 84, 104
endothelium, 73
endurance, 108
energy, 35, 36, 38
England, 79, 117, 123
enkephalins, 74, 84
entrapment, 37, 38
environment, 23, 35, 145, 147, 148, 149
epidural abscess, 101, 102, 103, 104, 117, 121, 129, 131, 132, 138
epinephrine, 124
equilibrium, 147
equipment, 4
ergonomics, viii, 17, 18, 19, 24, 26, 27, 30, 31, 32
esophagus, 48
ESR, 104
etanercept, 93, 118, 124, 130, 133, 141
European Commission, 147, 156
evidence, vii, viii, x, 1, 3, 6, 7, 10, 11, 14, 17, 19, 30, 34, 39, 79, 87, 95, 96, 99, 103, 105, 106, 112, 118, 119, 122, 127, 143, 146, 147, 150, 151, 152, 153, 155
evolution, 113, 158
excitability, 75, 78, 139
excitation, 77, 88
exercise, 20, 25, 27, 70, 71, 94, 107, 108, 114, 118, 127, 147, 153, 158
exertion, 148
experimental condition, ix, x, 57, 58, 59, 60, 61, 62, 63, 64, 65, 66
experimental design, 66, 149
experts, 91
exposure, 5
extensor, 77, 89
external environment, 149
extracts, 111, 123, 128, 136
extravasation, 73

F

factor analysis, 151
failure, 90
fainting, 145
false negative, 97

families, 84
family, 74, 80, 87, 137
fascia, viii, 33, 34, 35, 36, 37, 38, 39, 46, 47, 48
fat, 47, 129, 130
Fata, 123
fatigue, 94, 110, 111
fatty acids, 79, 110, 121
FDA, 83, 89, 98, 100, 101
fear, x, 143, 145, 148, 150, 151, 152, 153, 155, 156, 157, 158
feedback, 149, 151
feelings, 25, 36, 148
females, 86
fever, 48, 49, 52, 53, 80, 83, 94, 129
fiber, 72, 75, 87, 90, 96, 119
fibers, 8, 35, 36, 38, 71, 72, 73, 75, 76, 84, 85, 98, 104, 124, 127, 130, 144, 145
fibroblasts, 39, 79, 107, 116, 138
fibromyalgia, 71, 92, 93, 105, 110, 111, 115, 119, 126, 129, 131, 135, 138
first-generation cephalosporin, 101, 103
fish, 110, 131, 134
fish oil, 110, 131
fitness, 38, 42
flavonol, 113
flexibility, 5, 38
flexor, 37, 108
flora, 52
fluid, 2, 48, 50, 77, 83, 87, 97, 102, 107, 130, 136, 137
focusing, 114, 148, 151
football, 25
force, ix, 3, 4, 18, 20, 35, 36, 37, 57, 58, 59, 64, 66
forebrain, 144
formation, 19, 30, 46, 80, 81, 89
fractures, 3, 52
France, 57, 59
free radicals, 77
frozen shoulder, viii, 33, 36
fungal infection, 103
fusion, 42, 86, 88, 93, 94, 122

G

GABA, 72, 76, 81, 92, 95, 101
gait, 37, 67, 148
ganglion, 9, 10, 11, 15, 73, 75, 76, 114, 123, 126, 132, 138, 139
gel, 95
gender, 114, 116
gender differences, 30, 31
gene, x, 69, 72, 73, 74, 75, 83, 116, 119, 122, 132, 133, 134, 135, 138, 141, 144

gene expression, 116, 119
generation, 76, 78, 107, 133, 144
genes, 74
genus, 87
geometry, 3
Germany, 31, 41
ginger, 128, 137
gingival, 49
ginseng, 112
gland, 47
glaucoma, 95
glia, 9
glutamate, 9, 10, 15, 72, 85, 127, 130, 144
glycine, 72, 76, 141
glycosaminoglycans, 109
gout, 107
grades, 114
grants, 12
gravitational field, 35
gravity, viii, 33, 35
gray matter, 150
grief, 144
groups, 96, 103, 135, 150
growth, 34, 72, 73, 78, 79, 103, 107, 122, 123, 129, 132
growth factor, 72, 73, 78, 79, 107, 122, 123, 129, 132
guidance, viii, 18, 19
guidelines, 34, 109, 128, 156, 157
gut, 74

H

half-life, 93
hands, 71, 150
harmful effects, x, 69
HE, 117
headache, 52, 70, 74, 77, 85, 88, 90, 92, 97, 98, 108, 115, 126, 142
healing, 39, 82, 106, 107, 113, 123, 146, 148
heart rate, 36, 37
heat, x, 69, 70, 84, 87, 96, 119, 139
height, ix, 21, 33, 59
helplessness, 152
hematoma, 99
hemophilia, 25
hepatotoxicity, 84
herbal medicine, 111, 133
heredity, 18
herniated, 70, 77, 97, 98
herniated nucleus pulposus, 97
heroin, 86, 123
heterogeneity, 146

hip, 109, 119, 130, 135
hip replacement, 130
hippocampus, 150
histamine, 72, 73, 77, 104, 113, 138
historical reason, 74
history, 41, 49, 59, 70, 97, 108, 146, 156
Hong Kong, 143, 153
hopes, 139, 148
hospice, 141
hospitalization, 84
hospitals, 113, 132, 153
hunting, 134
hybridization, 141
hydrogen, 77
hydrogen peroxide, 77
hydroxyl, 77
hyoid, 47
hyperhidrosis, 89
hypersensitivity, vii, 2, 10, 11, 72, 80, 94, 95, 131, 132, 144
hypertension, 12
hypnosis, 106
hypothalamus, 150
hypothesis, viii, ix, 2, 3, 4, 5, 6, 12, 33, 140

I

ibuprofen, 83, 93, 120, 132, 138
identification, xi, 51, 144, 153
idiopathic, 97
IL-6, 72, 109, 112, 138
IL-8, 72, 138
iliopsoas, 37
image, 50
imagery, 106
images, 150
immune function, 85
immune response, 93
immune system, 78
immunocompromised, 49
immunodeficiency, 107
immunohistochemistry, 11
immunoreactivity, 115, 126
impacts, 153
impairments, xi, 37, 39, 41, 143, 146, 153
impregnation, 8
improvements, 36, 37, 93
impulses, 76, 77, 78, 81
in situ hybridization, 141
in vitro, 4, 110, 112, 113, 116, 117, 119, 123, 125, 127, 135, 136, 138, 140
in vivo, 6, 7, 14, 36, 122, 128
incidence, 10, 46, 52, 70, 104

independent variable, 20, 26
India, 112, 113
indication, 101
individuals, 35, 39, 70, 86, 89, 108, 114, 140
induction, 133
industry, 19
infants, 56
infliximab, 93
informed consent, 59
ingredients, 113, 141
initiation, 79
injections, x, 2, 69, 79, 89, 92, 97, 98, 99, 107, 115, 119, 121, 122, 128, 129, 132
insomnia, 90, 97
instinct, 151
Instron, 4
instruments, 113, 128
insulin, 137
integration, vii, 32, 34, 35, 36, 37, 42, 43, 139, 146
integrity, viii, 33, 35, 36, 101, 108, 110
interface, 50
interference, 51, 89
interferon, 73
interleukins, 73
internal consistency, 151, 152
intervention, vii, x, 32, 34, 41, 51, 69, 147, 148, 157
intramuscular injection, 89
intravenous drug abusers, 86
intravenously, 79, 103
ion channels, 78, 79, 87
ionizing radiation, 50
ions, 106
Iowa, 14, 34
ipsilateral, 5
ischemia, 94
issues, 126

J

Japan, 45
jaw, 132
joint pain, vii, 1, 2, 6, 11, 12, 85, 94, 97, 107, 112, 130, 131, 132
joints, vii, viii, 1, 2, 3, 5, 6, 11, 12, 13, 14, 15, 18, 37, 38, 87, 97, 108, 125
Jordan, 108, 109, 127, 147, 156
juvenile rheumatoid arthritis, 93

K

kinetics, 79
knee arthroplasty, 130

knots, 36
kyphosis, 89, 125

L

laboratory studies, 34
laminectomy, 97
laptop, 22
latency, 95, 135
lattices, 39
lead, ix, 7, 34, 39, 40, 41, 45, 53, 71, 74, 76, 78, 96, 105, 113, 148, 149
learning, 67
lesions, vii, ix, 2, 13, 45, 53, 83
leukotrienes, 78, 79
lifestyle, 147
ligament, 2, 5, 7, 9, 14, 46, 72, 107, 122, 123
ligand, 76, 77, 85
light, 103
likelihood, xi, 144
limbic system, 145
limitation, 83
line, 92
links, 93
lipids, 80, 109
liver, 107, 110
liver disease, 110
local anesthesia, 51
local anesthetic, x, 2, 69, 90, 97, 98, 100, 107, 124, 128
localization, 51, 72, 116, 131
locomotor, 119
locus, 58, 66
longitudinal study, 155
lumbar spine, 156
lymph, 46, 47, 49, 52
lymph node, 46, 47, 49, 52
lymphocytes, 72, 73

M

macrophages, 72, 73, 79, 93
magnesium, 76
magnet, 106
magnets, 106, 109, 125
magnitude, 7, 10, 36, 40
maintenance, 133
majority, 21, 23, 24, 80, 86
malignancy, 70
mammals, 74, 75
man, 77, 91, 134, 140

management, vii, x, xi, 38, 42, 46, 51, 52, 53, 54, 55, 56, 69, 80, 93, 95, 105, 106, 108, 110, 115, 116, 125, 126, 127, 128, 130, 135, 136, 141, 143, 144, 146, 147, 148, 153, 155, 156, 157
mandible, 47
manipulation, 34, 36, 37, 39, 42, 104, 107, 108, 114, 118, 121, 126, 127, 133, 137, 139, 146, 147, 156
mapping, 150
market, 83
marketing, 21
marrow, 136
mass, 3, 50
masseter, 47
mast cells, 72, 73, 78
materials, 106
matrix, 36, 79, 109, 115, 122, 127, 138
matrix metalloproteinase, 79, 115, 122, 127, 138
meanings, 145
measurements, 5, 7, 151
measures, xi, 71, 110, 143, 151, 153
mediastinitis, 46, 49, 50, 55
mediastinum, ix, 45, 48, 49, 51
mediation, 106
Mediterranean, 17, 21
membranes, 81, 110, 131
men, xi, 70, 114, 125, 144
mental state, 36
meta-analysis, 36, 109, 116, 136, 142, 155
metabolism, 95, 110, 111, 112, 113
metabolites, 72, 78, 84, 137
metalloproteinase, 79, 110, 122, 138
metastasis, 53
metatarsal, 65
meter, 123
methyl group, 110
methylprednisolone, 98, 99
mice, 73, 77, 119, 121, 123, 126, 128, 130, 141
microcirculation, 39
microorganisms, 48, 101
migraine headache, 74
migration, 79, 93, 107
mind-body, 41
miniature, 14
mobility, 106, 109, 111, 113, 114
model, x, 75, 82, 83, 84, 92, 94, 96, 103, 111, 120, 124, 129, 131, 132, 133, 137, 138, 141, 143, 146, 147, 148, 153, 157, 158
models, 7, 27, 32, 41, 74, 83, 85, 95, 139
modern society, xi, 144
mood, 86, 110
morbidity, 46

morphine, 71, 73, 74, 76, 85, 86, 91, 92, 95, 97, 98, 100, 101, 111, 116, 120, 125, 131, 133, 136, 138, 140, 141
morphology, 9
mortality, 46, 49, 98
mortality rate, 49, 98
motion, 82, 89, 103, 116, 156
motor behavior, 149
motor control, 58, 108, 126
motor neurons, 90
movement, 39, 70, 77, 88, 105, 108, 151, 153, 158
MRI, 51, 155
mRNA, 9, 129
mRNAs, 74, 76, 116
mucous membrane, 48
multidimensional, 39, 41
multiple sclerosis, 90, 95
muscarinic receptor, 95
musculoskeletal system, 18

N

necrosis, x, 69, 73, 93, 124, 130, 141
necrotizing fasciitis, 54
Netherlands, xi, 135, 144, 155
network, 145, 151
neural function, 92
neuralgia, 71, 87, 88, 92, 96, 99, 140
neutral, 5, 24, 60, 67
neutrophils, 72
Nigeria, 124
nightmares, 97
nitric oxide, 72, 73, 76, 77, 109, 110, 111, 126, 127, 137
nitric oxide synthase, 76
nitrogen, 77
NMDA receptors, 76, 91
N-methyl-D-aspartic acid, 141
Nobel Prize, 80
non-steroidal anti-inflammatory drugs, 92, 132, 137
norepinephrine, 77, 92
North America, 42, 54, 135
NSAIDs, 80, 81, 82, 83, 84, 91, 125, 135, 140, 146
nuclei, 150
nucleus, 97, 127, 133, 137, 144
nurses, xi, 31, 144, 158
nutrients, 37, 38

O

obstruction, 46, 49, 53
odynophagia, 48
oedema, 119
oil, 107, 110, 112, 113, 129, 131
old age, 35
omega-3, 79, 110, 116, 137
one dimension, 39
opiates, 95
opioids, 72, 74, 76, 86, 100, 125, 127, 128, 139
opportunities, 94
order, 84, 91, 144, 145, 146, 148, 151, 153
organ, 35, 40
organism, 53, 103
organs, 35, 70, 79, 94
osteoarthritis, 70, 75, 79, 83, 84, 88, 95, 107, 109, 110, 111, 112, 117, 119, 120, 122, 123, 126, 127, 129, 132, 133, 134, 135, 136, 139, 141, 142
osteomyelitis, 52, 56, 70, 86, 101, 102, 103, 116, 118, 121, 122, 123, 127, 130, 132, 136, 138
osteopathy, 34
ovarian cancer, 130
overtime, 71
oxygen, 77

P

palpation, 105
parallel, 86, 139, 151
paralysis, 123
parameters, 90, 120
parotid, 47, 53
parotid duct, 47
parotid gland, 47
participants, ix, 21, 57, 58, 59, 60, 61, 64, 66, 106, 107
particles, 99
partition, 101
passive, 108
patents, 118
pathogenesis, 74, 105
pathogens, 51, 101
pathology, 40, 58, 71, 146, 148
pathophysiological, 80
pathophysiology, 38
pathways, x, 7, 40, 78, 84, 90, 111, 113, 128, 131, 137, 143, 144, 145, 146, 147, 150
pelvis, 35, 37
penicillin, 51, 103
peptide, x, 3, 11, 12, 15, 69, 72, 73, 74, 75, 100, 122, 132, 133, 134, 135, 138, 141, 144
peptides, 72, 73, 74, 76, 80, 84
perceptions, 157
perceptual component, 40
performance, 105, 151
perfusion, 142

Index

periodontal, 55, 112, 136
periodontal disease, 55
peripheral neuropathy, 87
permit, 106
peroxide, 77
personality, 39
PET, 150
pH, 79, 101, 106, 138
phantom limb pain, 91, 141
pharmaceutical, 82, 115
pharmacology, 122
pharmacotherapy, x, 69
pharyngitis, 52, 54
pharynx, 48
phenol, 107
Philadelphia, 42, 132, 135, 139, 146, 157
phospholipids, 110
phosphorylation, 81
photographs, ix, 33
photomicrographs, 8
physical activity, 41, 91, 151
physical environment, 147
physical health, 18
physical therapist, ix, 34, 38, 41, 42
physical therapy, viii, x, 33, 34, 43, 69, 114
physiological mechanisms, 148
physiology, 38, 40, 120, 156
pilot study, 123, 124, 131
placebo, 84, 89, 90, 91, 92, 93, 96, 111, 112, 120, 121, 123, 126, 129, 130, 131, 132, 134, 135, 136, 139, 141
planning, xi, 144
plants, x, 69, 87, 110, 113
plasma, 73, 139
plasma membrane, 139
plastic surgeon, 36
plasticity, vii, 2, 10, 11, 15, 42, 126
platelet aggregation, 84
platelets, 72, 80
platform, ix, 57, 58, 59, 64, 66
platysma, 47
playing, 110
pleural effusion, 50
plexus, 117, 124
PM, 129, 139, 142, 156
point of origin, 40
policy, 156
polyamines, 81
polymerase, 121
polymerase chain reaction, 121
polypeptide, 115, 116, 138
polyps, 83
poor, 98, 104, 114

population, x, xi, 25, 70, 71, 114, 116, 121, 123, 143, 144, 155, 156
positrons, 150
postural control, ix, 57, 58, 63, 64, 65, 66, 67, 149
posture, 148
potassium, 72, 75, 100
prediction, 157
predictor variables, viii, 17
predictors, 153
pregnancy, 18
preparation, 77, 82, 90, 110, 111, 113, 115
pressure, 77, 105, 106, 108, 121, 125
prevention, 30, 32, 104
primate, 149
principles, 128
private practice, 33
problem-solving, 43
production, 73, 74, 77, 78, 79, 80, 81, 82, 89, 106, 110, 112, 113, 117, 128, 137, 138, 140
professionals, 40
program, 108, 114, 125, 127, 157
project, 144
proliferation, 110, 124
properties, 74, 79, 82, 90, 98, 110, 112, 113, 116, 123, 127, 148, 158
prophylactic, 102, 103, 134
prophylaxis, 139
proposition, 6
prostaglandins, 72, 77, 78, 80, 81, 83, 84, 105, 110, 111, 112, 113, 136
prostate, 134
protection, 4, 80
protein kinase C, 10, 15, 77
protein synthesis, 82
proteins, 80, 93, 109
proteoglycans, 109, 124
proteolytic enzyme, 109, 119
protocol, 106
psoriasis, 93
psoriatic arthritis, 93
psychological well-being, 34
psychologist, 156
psychosocial factors, x, 143, 147, 148, 153
psychotherapy, 36
pumps, 101
puncture wounds, 52
punishment, 144
purines, 77, 136
P-value, 29
pyogenic, 122, 125

Q

quality of life, x, xi, 69, 85, 98, 105, 107, 113, 114, 118, 133, 136, 144
quantification, 66, 123
quercetin, 113, 127, 134
questionnaire, viii, 17, 19, 20, 21, 23, 37, 113, 114, 151, 152, 157, 158

R

race, 101
radiation, 150
Radiation, 41
radicals, 77
radiculopathy, 70, 77, 98, 119, 125, 128, 129, 132
radiography, 12, 50
range, 70, 76, 86, 89, 103, 105, 106, 108, 117, 119, 146, 153, 156
rash, 83, 94
rating scale, 152, 153
ratio analysis, 27
reactions, 72, 83, 95, 97, 98, 100, 110, 111, 128
reactivity, 158
reading, 155
receptive field, 40
receptors, viii, 2, 6, 7, 8, 12, 14, 37, 38, 71, 72, 74, 75, 76, 77, 78, 84, 91, 93, 94, 95, 96, 98, 100, 118, 122, 127, 130, 131, 132, 135, 136, 142
recombinant DNA, 94
recommendations, iv, 102, 109
reconstruction, 122
recreation, xi, 144
red blood cells, 99
redistribution, 37, 38
reflex sympathetic dystrophy, 140
reflexes, 8, 71, 73, 92
regeneration, 3, 107, 126
region, 70, 88, 107
regulation, 75, 76, 79, 84, 119, 127
rehabilitation, xi, 42, 43, 105, 107, 114, 144, 147, 153, 156, 157
rehabilitation program, 114, 147, 153
relationship, 147, 150, 153
relaxation, 39, 106, 125
relevance, 19, 129
reliability, 50, 67, 146, 151, 152
relief, 2, 3, 71, 85, 86, 87, 95, 97, 98, 99, 100, 105, 107, 108, 113, 114, 115, 122, 126
repair, 79, 107
repetitions, 108
replication, 106

requirements, 18, 90, 133
researchers, 4, 34, 37, 39, 149
residuals, 26
resistance, 54, 89, 109
resolution, 40, 41, 50, 51, 53, 79, 137
resources, ix, 58, 65
respect, x, 69
respiratory, 99, 100
respiratory arrest, 99
response, vii, 2, 6, 7, 10, 11, 14, 40, 41, 52, 71, 73, 75, 76, 81, 87, 89, 90, 91, 93, 94, 97, 98, 99, 105, 120, 128, 133, 139, 145, 147, 150, 152
response behaviors, 150
responsiveness, 74, 89, 152
restoration, 37, 38, 71, 108
restrictions, 70
resveratrol, 137
rheumatic diseases, 125, 128, 131
rheumatoid arthritis, 25, 73, 79, 83, 87, 93, 94, 95, 106, 107, 110, 112, 116, 121, 125, 129, 140
rhizome, 128
RNA, 74, 110, 116
root, 9, 10, 11, 15, 67, 75, 76, 79, 97, 112, 114, 117, 118, 123, 126, 132, 137, 138, 139, 144, 145
rotations, 4

S

safety, 117, 125, 132
salivary gland, 47, 48
scaling, 7
school, 114
sciatica, 93, 98, 124
science, 41, 42
sclerosis, 90, 95
scores, 83, 96, 105, 113, 114, 125, 151, 153
screening, 123
secrete, 75
secretion, 104
sedative, 90, 113
sedatives, 92
seed, 112, 129
selectivity, 85
self-regulation, 127
sensation, 39, 41, 70, 73, 76, 80, 87, 119, 138, 145
sensations, 39, 40, 144, 152
sensing, 79, 140
sensitivity, 10, 51, 71, 74, 76, 79, 103, 105, 106, 117
sensitization, 7, 11, 72, 73, 77, 78, 81, 85, 117, 120, 124
separation, 88
sepsis, ix, 45, 46, 52, 54, 55, 103
septic arthritis, 53, 123

septic discitis, 103
septic shock, 49
serotonin, 72, 73, 81, 84, 104, 105, 118, 136
serum, 77, 102, 129
services, iv, 41
severity, 71, 85, 88, 146
sexual behavior, 122
shape, 8, 35
shares, 93
shear, 3, 4, 5, 14
shock, 49
shoulders, 107, 114
showing, viii, 11, 33
sickle cell, 129
side effects, 78, 86, 97, 100, 136
signal transduction, 81
signals, 6, 35, 39, 78, 137, 145, 151
significance level, 20
signs, 13, 48, 103, 112
silver, 8
simulations, 5
sinuses, 48
skeletal muscle, 90, 105, 137
skills, 114
skin, 36, 38, 39, 42, 53, 73, 83, 95, 98, 106, 124, 134, 138
skull fracture, 13
smoking, 23
smooth muscle, 78
social activities, 149
social class, 116
social interactions, 147
society, xi, 144
socioeconomic background, 145
sodium, 79, 83, 92, 117, 123, 128
software, 60
solution, 38, 90, 96, 107
soybean, 123
space, 86, 97, 101, 102, 108, 141
spasticity, 90, 92, 98, 101, 116, 139
species, 49, 77, 101, 103, 149
spectrum, 103, 141
spine, vii, ix, 2, 3, 4, 5, 6, 8, 11, 13, 14, 34, 38, 43, 46, 48, 52, 70, 85, 86, 93, 97, 99, 100, 101, 103, 112, 114, 118, 119, 126, 130, 135, 137, 139, 140, 141, 156
spore, 88
sprains, 71, 72, 87, 107
stability, 2, 35, 60, 66, 67
stabilization, 147
standard error, 62, 63, 64, 65
staphylococci, 102, 120, 128
state, 35, 36, 37, 42, 71, 72, 76, 129

states, 35, 38, 39, 74, 115, 122
stenosis, 97, 98, 107
steroids, x, 69, 97, 98, 107, 111, 112, 129
stimulus, 10, 39, 40, 59, 107, 118, 119, 144, 145, 150, 151, 155
stomach, 80, 111
strabismus, 89
strain, 70, 90, 95, 99
strategies, 114, 115, 147
strategy, 106, 129, 148
strength, 85, 106, 111, 112, 117, 156
strength training, 117
streptococci, 49, 52, 102
stress, 35, 36, 37, 45, 94, 114
stretching, 9, 14, 38, 70, 147
stroke, 90
structural changes, 36
structure, 35, 36, 38, 40, 42, 107, 109, 119, 132
subacute, 147, 148
subgroups, 137, 140
substance use, 86
success rate, 105
sugar, 109
sulfate, 101, 109, 110, 117, 119, 120, 122, 134
summer, 112
supervisor, 23
supplementation, 110
suppression, 87, 88, 93, 97, 113, 140
surface area, 60, 62, 64
survey, 84, 114, 152
susceptibility, 54
swelling, 24, 39, 48, 49, 51, 52, 53, 97
switching, 117
symmetry, 36
sympathetic nervous system, 37, 77, 78
synaptic transmission, 142
syndrome, 2, 32, 40, 52, 53, 54, 55, 67, 70, 71, 85, 88, 89, 92, 94, 97, 99, 100, 101, 105, 118, 123, 124, 129, 134, 138, 146, 149
synergistic effect, 93
synthesis, 81, 82, 83, 84, 98, 109, 110, 113, 122, 124, 131, 138

T

T cell, 112, 131
tar, 83
techniques, viii, 33, 34, 36, 136, 150, 151
technology, 94
teeth, 48, 49, 50
teicoplanin, 103
temperature, 36, 79, 87, 94
tendon, 82, 107, 116, 125

tendons, 18, 35, 37, 38, 71, 107
tension, 32, 35, 37, 38, 90, 92, 105
tension headache, 90, 92
terminals, 76, 79, 80, 85, 92, 100
testing, 6
test-retest reliability, 60, 61, 152
textbook, 157
thalamus, 95, 127, 144, 145
therapeutic agents, 119
therapeutic interventions, 9, 34
therapeutic use, 95, 125
therapists, 137, 149
therapy, viii, x, 33, 35, 36, 38, 46, 53, 69, 85, 86, 89, 90, 92, 93, 97, 102, 103, 104, 105, 106, 107, 109, 111, 112, 114, 116, 120, 124, 126, 127, 128, 129, 136, 137, 146, 153, 158
thorax, 35
thrombophlebitis, 53, 54, 55
thrombosis, 46, 49, 51, 56
thromboxanes, 78
thyroid, 25, 48
timing, 148
tin, 24
tissue, vii, viii, 2, 7, 9, 10, 11, 13, 33, 34, 35, 36, 37, 38, 39, 40, 42, 50, 52, 54, 71, 72, 74, 77, 79, 82, 87, 101, 103, 107, 112, 122, 129, 135, 138, 145, 146, 147, 148
tonic, 89, 94
tonsils, 48, 49
tooth, 52, 55, 142
tooth abscess, 55
torsion, 89
torticollis, 55, 88
total energy, 7
toxicity, 83
toxin, 87, 88, 89, 92, 115, 118, 119, 120, 123, 125, 128, 134, 135, 139, 141
training, 34, 108, 117, 127, 151, 153, 156
trajectory, 60, 62
transcripts, 74
transduction, 81
transection, 127
transformation, 137
transforming growth factor, 79
translation, 152
transmission, 40, 73, 76, 77, 78, 79, 81, 95, 100, 128, 142, 146
transport, 10, 11, 90, 118, 122
transportation, 79
trapezius, 27, 77, 98
trauma, 30, 35, 49, 71, 81, 104, 105
tremor, 88

trial, 38, 60, 61, 83, 90, 91, 117, 118, 120, 121, 123, 124, 126, 127, 130, 133, 134, 136, 138, 140, 141, 146, 155, 156
tricyclic antidepressant, 93, 96
tricyclic antidepressants, 93
trigeminal nerve, 47
trigeminal neuralgia, 88, 92
triggers, 79
tuberculosis, 52, 121
tumor, x, 47, 69, 73, 93, 113, 130, 141
tumor necrosis factor, x, 69, 73, 93, 130, 141

U

ultrasound, 39, 50, 114, 134, 146
uniform, 9, 99
upper respiratory tract, 54
uric acid, 113

V

validation, 27, 67, 158
valuation, 54
vancomycin, 102, 103, 120
variables, x, 60, 61, 143, 148
variance, 152
varicose veins, 36
varieties, 113
vasoactive intestinal peptide, 73
vasoconstriction, 90
vasodilator, 74, 142
vasomotor, 87
vegetables, 113
vein, 46, 47, 49, 51, 53, 54, 55
velocity, 13, 37, 60, 62, 63, 64
venlafaxine, 118
ventricle, 142, 150
vertebrae, vii, ix, 4, 13, 24, 45, 48, 52, 149
vertebral artery, 48, 97
vertigo, 66
vesicle, 88
vessels, 8, 37, 47, 50
vibration, 42
victims, 13
volleyball, 25

W

walking, 25, 155
war, 35
Washington, 136

waste, 37, 38
water, 101
weakness, 24, 36, 86, 89, 107
web, 21
wind, 85, 91
withdrawal, 95, 116, 149
women, xi, 70, 114, 125, 144
worldwide, x, 69, 83

Y

yield, 7, 14, 98
young adults, 53, 66
young people, 38

Z

zinc, 136